THE DYNAMICS OF WORLD CLASS FOOTBALL-SOCCER

NEWTONIAN FOOTBALL – SOCCER TRAINING AND PLAYING MANUAL

James J Lall Petro., Chem., Engineer

WORLD CLASS FOOTBALL-SOCCER LTD
www.dynamicsoffootballsoccer.co.uk

I would like to dedicate this book to my wife Deirdre, and children Sharon, David, and Debbie.

Edited by World Class Football-Soccer Ltd

Published by World Class Football-Soccer Ltd

A catalogue record of this book is available at the British Library

ISBN 978-178035-441-5

Printed and bound in the UK

Preface

The football / soccer players who read this manual seeks perfection - those who implement its ideas have found it. This inspirational world class training, and playing football / soccer manual uses a designed, and developed pragmatic approach in the analysis, and solution of unsteady state football / soccer phenomenon - in conjunction with chosen basic engineering fluid and particle dynamics principles incorporating Analogies, with mental psychology for CONTROLLING the game - and shows how they are all interconnected.
This manual transcends imagination and originality.
Simple to follow the manual converge on the systems in harmony as one unit, shows how the experience of the coach, in relation to the player, and team-mates relate for discipline on and off the pitch, and accomplish learning.

Bring into sharp focus those fine points, which enable the players to apply the fundamental principles correctly, confidently, consistently, and with continuity - for example, Newton's laws for complete body and ball control.
A qualitative, and quantitative understanding of the application of the principles to realistic problems in training and playing are particularly emphasised. It guides the players into forming organised patterns of defence, and attack - DEFINES THE DEFINING MOMENT IN DEFENCE: and THE DEFINING MOMENT OF THE FINAL BALL.
Helps the players to develop character, and to achieve the ability to "GEL" together to play good exciting free flowing attacking NEWTONIAN football - soccer with breath-taking displays: beautiful at its most intense: played in the TRUE SPIRIT of the system – a thing of beauty is joy forever.
This unique brand of Newtonian football/soccer the players likes to play, and and the fans likes to watch – the right way how football/soccer should be played: always wanting more of the same.

Numerous simple mathematical examples are worked out in detail to illustrate some of the basic principles that are discussed for mental awareness.
A good genuine, solid base with four different exciting styles to train, and to play from - and when things go wrong - and sometimes they do from the the smallest problem to the chaotic and dysfunctional - the enigma wrapped in a nightmare scenario – make the invisible visible, and how to put them right.
Implementation of the system during training, and playing for a number of months will transform the players, and team from the ordinary to the sublime with optimum performance. Revenue and crowd capacity goes up.
The system has been proven during, and after the development stages over a number of years, at all levels of football /soccer from World Cup - English premiership and lower divisions, and this manual is the world's first of its kind, and sets the ultimate standard to aim for. This brand of football-soccer will not be surpassed due to the laws of nature and will be played forever.
This manual is intended for people of all background, who are interested in enhancing, and furthering their football /soccer career.
Suitable for coaches, managers, men and women footballers, secondary schools and upwards - football / soccer fans - giving excitement, and happiness to players: and spectators alike. I would like to thank some of the coaches and managers for their trials in making this manual possible.

James J Lall

Belief

If you do what is right believe in what you do, and do it well. Football is about opinions and views. Some people have opinions and views of the game and how it should be played. For a system to work it must be backed up by facts and the truth. If it does not work, it is not a system, whether it is closed or open, football must be kept simple in the players mind. You are trying to score, and the opponent is trying to stop you and vice-versa, the winner will have the better ideas and makes the least mistakes. The individual or gifted players will make a difference, but basically football is a team effort - reading from one book.

Mistakes will be made, even with the best training preparation by coaches - players - teams etc., put this down to human error, that spur of the moment decision - which is indefinable and mysterious - and since we cannot control, comprehend or explain this is where divine intervention is sought.
The LORD instils in ordinary people the ability to do extraordinary things. Miracles do happen - it has been proved many times over.
When a person comes to JESUS and does the things JESUS says – this is like a person who dug deep and built a house on solid rock: when the rain and flood beat against the house - the house held firm and did not fall down, because it was built on solid foundation. The person who did not come to JESUS, and did not do the things JESUS said, built a house on sandy earth - when the rain and flood came the house fell down, because it was not built on solid foundation. A good tree produces good fruits, and a bad tree produces bad fruits. Out of a good heart comes good things, and out of a bad heart comes bad things.

JESUS is the beautiful light of the world.
When JESUS was a little boy he played ball games with his siblings, so he knows about football long before us - he also knows how the game will turn out, because he knows exactly what every player is thinking.
A little prayer, said before or during the game helps - sometimes directly, sometimes indirectly, and with the LORD and MASTER on your side you cannot go wrong. JESUS said, seek and ye shall find - knock and it shall be opened - ask and it shall be given - THINK before you say or do anything - boast not of tomorrow, for one knows not what tomorrow brings - focus on today, for today's troubles are more than enough - then think of tomorrow: take one day at a time - the TRUTH. Glory in tribulations knowing that from tribulations comes patience, and from patience comes experience, and from experience comes hope, and from hope not to be ashamed. Rejoice in the hope of the glory of God, because the love of GOD is shed abroad in our hearts by the HOLY GHOST which is given unto us.

Belief

In religion - the word of the LORD is the truth. For we can do nothing against the truth, but for the TRUTH. We must not lie against the TRUTH because there is no lie in the TRUTH.
If you score three goals and the opponent score one - you will win.
In mathematics - four plus three equals seven is the truth.
In general the truth is the only correct answer - that is the beauty of the truth. Seek the truth for only from the truth you will be able to tell RIGHT from WRONG and when something is wrong you speak out – you do not leave it or ignore it – you fix it.
If someone does you harm in any way or form, do not seek revenge - for then there are no come-backs. The HOLY TRINITY decides.
JESUS said obey the commandments, these would help you to maintain moral discipline where right and wrong is concerned. Avoid hypocrisy.

JESUS has taught us great things, and those great things are backed up by great deeds he has done and is doing today. Deeds such as love, how to help the poor, charity, healing, compassion, forgiveness, humility – how to remember, right from wrong – the sanctity of marriage between a man and a woman. How to avoid being greedy. What does it profit a man to win the world, and then lose himself. How to understand by listening, reading and remembering using interest and concentration as your focus. How to sit down and work out problems mathematically or otherwise to get the right solutions - how to use common sense - and priority at times.
How not to bear false witness against thy neighbour and how to live in harmony: protect children from abuse and harm, and how to be a family.
For life and peace it is better to be more spiritually minded than carnally minded with an inclination to edification.
How to avoid idle talk and foolishness: when and where to draw the line.
Ask and teach a small child what CHRISTMAS is about - and the answer should be about JESUS, his teachings - gifts, food, and fun in that order from a young age.
JESUS said, there is no greater gift than LOVE – love the HOLY TRINITY- and love one another as I have loved you. JESUS said believe in me and I will send you a COMFORTER forever. Let not then your good be evil spoken of: a double minded man is unstable in all his ways.
Give credit where credit is due: for the kingdom of God is not meat and drink; but righteousness, and peace, and joy in the HOLY GHOST.
WEAR THE BELT OF TRUTH - THE BREAST- PLATE OF RIGHTEOUSNESS - AND THE SWORD OF THE SPIRIT THESE ARE THE WORDS OF GOD.
Without ambiguity stay out of trouble - live a good life, and set good examples for others to follow. This is up to you, if you read one page a day or one page a week of the new testament the BEST BOOK in the world, there is so much to learn you will find it very fulfilling and rewarding – and help to make this world a safer, and better place for generations to come.

Contents Page

Contents Page

Contents Page

Contents Page

Contents Page

CHEATING

Cheating goes on at various levels within the population by some people in marriage, education, jobs, sports and takes various forms such as fraud, lying, corruption, match-fixing, deception and hypocrisy. These are bad things and should not enter your thoughts.
When rules and laws are made to live, play, and work by there is always a crook willing to break it, in order to create an unfair advantage at the expense of someone else or the opponent.
There are some people who will do wrong and swear it is right, and some people will tell you a blatant lie, to get what they want and say it is the truth - these people have no shame what so ever. They cannot be trusted. Nothing good comes out of lies.

Cheating is a temptation to violate the rules or do wrong – at times it could be a deliberate act, and sometimes it could be a spur of the moment thing. Think of the consequences and avoid making this type of mistake.
In football – soccer cheating can take many forms such as deceiving the referee – deliberate handling of the ball, and hope the referee does not see the incident.
Deliberate diving or going down too easily to gain a penalty is a form of cheating.
Some players will stoop quite low to apply direct and indirect cheating tactics in the opponent penalty area, by way of placing their foot around an opponent leg, so as to trip-up to gain a penalty.
Deliberate faking injury to increase playing stoppage time which gives them a few extra minutes to level the score or win the game, and this makes it difficult for the opponent to strike back.
Some players get opponent yellow carded or red carded and sent off, so that the opponent becomes weaker to gain an unfair advantage.
Provocation by opponents is another form of cheating - especially if one or more of your team-mates are sent off – this weakens the team and disrupts the game plan – it is important that players do not fall for these tricks. Deliberate kicking or hitting an opponent, and he/she has to go off the pitch, while play goes on is another form of cheating.
In some cases players who used to play for previous teams tend to have a soft spot for that team, and does not like scoring against them – it is a form of cheating, but difficult to prove.
Some players fake injury to avoid training sessions – this does not help the team.
Some cheating incidents are difficult to prove at any point in time, but slow motion cameras can solve some of them, and show right from wrong.
If you value your moral behaviour, character, integrity, and dignity you will not cheat.
Try to resist the urge to cheat then there will be no comebacks, because cheating tactics are no good, and they are not right – SO DON'T DO IT.

Chapter 1

Health and Fitness

Health and fitness are the most important departments in life in general, and football in particular; having the senses, emotion and minds under control - you are now able to focus one hundred percent on football-soccer. There is a significant amount of interest attached to health and fitness, for the benefit of leisure and games. Coaches and managers have recognised the importance of physical exercises. Since benefits are achieved from physical exercise, they also, extend to the emotional and mental aspects of the players.

Physical exercise helps to control weight, reduces tension, stiffness, improves health, and also helps to solve emotional problems. For a footballer safe cardiovascular exercises are important for health and fitness. With all exercises, players have their limitations and injury should be avoided at all cost, for example, regular heading of high velocity balls coming in from crosses can cause brain damage – see Impact and Impulse in Chapter 5. There is an optimum standard where a player's limitations are of concern, with various exercises such as velocity, and acceleration in running, stretching, leaping etc, when the standard is reached, the player will not improve any further, because in trying to exceed the optimum standard injury may occur.

Strength: Stamina: Speed requires control.

Strength: to be strong - no pushover - up to the mark - and mentally focused.

Stamina: to last the distance – able to play for ninety minutes plus extra time and out-stay the opponent.

Speed: to be fast – able to out-run and out-stay the opponent within reason.

Calories and Energy- the amount of heat to change temp- 1gm of water by 1degree C

When a footballer plays for ninety minutes plus extra time, he has done an amount of work. The footballer was fed, and his/ her food was turned into fuel. The chemical energy of the food can be measured, if a small quantity of it is burnt. Adding together, the heat value of the work, and the heat that the footballer's body gives off - this gives the total chemical energy of the food the footballer consumed. The number of calories a footballer needs is a minimum of 3000 to 3500 calories per day. The footballer may use the numbers as a guide for his/her daily intake - and with the doctor, and dietician advice chooses a suitable quantity of calories intake per day. A trial and error method could be used, to get this right, depending on the footballer's height and weight.
Muscles have a special quality in turning chemical energy into mechanical energy. When the muscles are working phosphates contained in the tissues, breaks down, and while this is happening, muscles fibres expands, and contracts through the bones, and joints – and the footballer's muscle does an amount of work - after contraction oxidation reactions of sugars, causes phosphates to accumulate to continue the cycle.

Sugar Level

If sugar is converted into energy, it must first enter the cells, to do this a key is needed to open the cells – this key is insulin, and is produced by the pancreas. To keep your sugar levels correct insulin is required to open the cells, so that sugar can enter the cells to be converted into energy. If for some reason the pancreas is not working properly, and cannot produce enough insulin dangerous levels of sugar will build up in the bloodstream which could lead to loss of energy, and damage to cells and vital organs in the body.

Blood Pressure –high or low salt level

Extremely important have it checked regularly, and to keep to a safe diet and salt intake balance.
To achieve free flowing circulation to the heart and lungs to keep them functioning at optimum level.

Hot And Humid Conditions –reduces salts- causes poor brain activity - giddiness

When football / soccer is trained or played in hot or humid conditions, footballers tend to lose body weight after each game – due to loss of body fluid, and essential salts such as sodium, and potassium through perspiration; as the perspiration dries these salt particles settles on the surface of the skin: loss of too much salts can cause players to suffer from cramp, and also affect the performance of the players. Milk contains lactic acid, and if, consumed in large quantities, can increase the risk of a cramp attack during a game.
If the body is very hot, and ice cold drinks are consumed quickly, this can cause severe stomach pain, and care should be taken to reduce this risk. Football / soccer is a fast game over a comparatively short period, and permitted fast energy release drinks should be taken during the game, and at half time, but be careful the temperature of the drink is not too low. Fizzy or carbonated drinks may also cause high acid/gas problems.

Stress

Sometimes stress is self-manifested – at other times it is inflicted by the opponent, and sometimes circumstances beyond anyone's control can cause stress. This is a serious problem for everyone concerned in general, and for coach, and players in particular: but if, you use the term – not who is right, but what is right – do what is right – and keep it right where mental and physical preparations are required for each game: when the optimum standard is reached, and maintained stress is usually kept to a minimum.
Stress is something we all have to cope with the best way we can at one time or another.

Training system – There are training systems sold on the market which helps players to develop greater leg power to the kicking foot – increase vertical leap – first step quickness – and reaction and response.

Warm up And Stretching

Before starting any stretching exercises for a football / soccer game, it is essential that the body be warmed up by light running or bike riding to reduce stiffness in the muscles, and ligaments, to increase blood circulation, and to avoid future damage to these parts.
When the body suffers from stiffness, tightness and tenseness – the body is not fully fit: relief is by mild stretching exercises. Stretching exercises should be done smoothly and slowly. Go as far as you can – but do not force to achieve extreme positions. The key is to hold the stretch for approximately 15 seconds – then slowly return to normal. The hold will gradually increase the elasticity that is needed to get the most extreme positions. Stretching exercises helps to keep the tissues of the muscles, ligaments, and tendons in good shape and maintain elasticity. Most injuries to players, are caused by their bodies not being flexible enough – that is, little or no elasticity. When players have to twist and turn, move quickly, awkwardly or stretch to some extreme to get the ball: it is at that moment enough elasticity must be within their bodies, so that difficult movements can be performed with a certain amount of ease, and keep injuries down to a minimum.
DO NOT OVERDO EXERCISES – YOU MUST GIVE THE BODY TIME TO RECOVER – the club physiotherapist and sport science personnel are best qualified to give help in this important field. Books in libraries and bookstores, are available on the subject, and players should attempt to read up and PERFECT PRACTICE the exercises, but take care when exercising.

The Kicking Foot

For a football / soccer player the kicking foot is the main armoury and needs a lot of care and attention. Most injuries to the kicking foot occur during training or playing – sometimes it is the players fault when he / she makes a mistake or mistimed a tackle or by a hard opponent. The worst damage is usually done when the player is not prepared for the collision as it happens unexpectedly. Most injuries on the pitch can be avoided, but requires the help of players involved – that is, team-mates and opponents alike.

When an opponent of a certain mass, and velocity collides with another player – depending on the line of action of the force unto the kicking foot – the momentum carried by the opponent produces a sudden impact which exceeds the elastic limit of an area of the bone, muscle or ligament within the kicking foot – this sudden impact creates a greater stress value, and although the sudden impact is only for a split second, it is at this point in time that serious damage occurs.

The applied force that causes the damage could be compressive, twist or spiral, bending or a tensile force. All three forces can cause serious damage to the kicking foot, if, the breaking point is exceeded.
The PELVIC or GROIN area contains bones, muscles, and tendons, and if, a player do not warm up – stretches beyond his / her limit or kicks the ground instead of the ball serious damage may occur to the pelvic area which could be a painful reality, and may take a long time to heal, and if not healed properly before resuming training could easily be aggravated, take even longer to heal: sometimes, if care is not taken could lead to permanent damage.

The kicking foot consists of the THIGH which is made up of the large bone called the FEMUR – attached to the femur are nerves, cartilage, tendons, and four muscles, which are called the hamstrings. Attached to the femur at the kneecap is the LEG BONE, which is made up of the TIBIA, and FIBULA and joined by ligaments, and covered by a layer of cartilage. The tibia is the larger bone, and the fibula is the smaller bone, the shin-bone is the front of the tibia, and can be felt as it lies under the skin.
The leg contains muscles, nerves, and tendons for attachment to the foot. The tibia and fibula are joined to the ankle by the cartilage to form the ankle joint. The foot consists of a number of muscles, ligaments, tendons and bones – and a number of bones called the TARSAL BONES. These bones are as follows – the TALUS bone is joined by the tibia, and fibula to form the ankle joint.
The HEELBONE or CALCANEUS is where the ACHILLES TENDON is attached. The CUBOID – NAVICULAR and the three CUNEIFORM bones makes up the other tarsal bones. At the sole of the foot are the METATARSAL bones, and the toe bones are called the PHALANGES.
The arch of the foot gives it strength, and act like a shock absorber for leaping and landing. The shape of the curve can vary from near flat to a considerable arch – ligaments, and tendons helps to keep the arch shape intact – damage to the metatarsal can be very painful, and takes a long time to heal due to the weight the foot has to carry: this also creates a weak spot in the foot for future collision. The ligaments at the ankle joint are the DELTOID, which connect vertically from the leg bone to the foot bone, and with three lateral ligaments known as the anterior talo-fibular, posterior talo-fibular, and the calcaneo-fibular ligaments.
Exceeding the elastic limit of these joints in any direction will result in serious damage.

Drugs and Alcohol abuse should not be tolerated in any event.

Food allergy – lactose intolerance – high and low blood sugar levels – high and low blood pressure, are some of the hidden dangers that can affect a player's health, and result in serious loss of energy. The doctor will be able to monitor, and take appropriate action to correct the problems. The footballer should read up on the complimentary therapy of REFLEXOLOGY – this is based on pressure points on the body in general, and the feet and hands in particular; it's a natural form of healing and energising the body, giving a feeling of well being. For good health, use foods and drinks that are 60/80% alkaline and 20/40% acid to give a precise blood pH value of 7.35 to 7.45. Poor health and fitness causes lack of energy. Lack of energy – means a player cannot perform with optimum efficiency for 90 minutes plus extra time: especially the last ten minutes of the game. So footballers must give health and fitness top priority in order to play well.

Chapter 2

Coach's Responsibilities

The coach or manager has two jobs – one his day-to-day Management, and dealing with club affairs – the other day-to-day Training ground Perfect Practice, which also includes health and fitness. With the help of this manual the coach or manager's job becomes less difficult. He can then concentrate on each job individually without becoming confused. His main priority is to produce GOOD EXCITING BEAUTIFUL FOOTBALL – SOCCER PREFERABLY KEEPING A CLEAN SHEET – GET GOOD RESULTS CONFIDENTLY, CONSISTENTLY, and CONTINOUSLY- and command the respect of the players.

Using his/her experience, in conjunction with the systems in this manual to help the players to complete the Perfect Practice called for. Use the training ground to get things right: iron out any problems mentally and physically. Allow players to express themselves in attack, on the training ground and on match days with a clean sheet in mind. Keep high morale and harmony within the team: maintain a high standard of play at home and away games. No sitting back at home or away games. Some coaches and players may, have covered certain aspects of fluid and particle dynamics at some stage; and this will give them a head start on others who have not done the subject before.
To the coaches and players who are new to the subject, will find it useful to work by implementing any of the styles you decide to play by given in Chapter 10 to start with: and then gradually weave piece by piece of the dynamics into the style of play. Do not try to do everything at once: take your time and Perfect Practice one thing at a time. Just by playing the styles, and using other information given in this manual: you can play some very good football; the dynamics helps to give you that extra edge of finer points to produce beautiful clever, wonderful, and breathtaking football with confidence, consistency and continuity.

Tinkering

At first, sometimes it will be necessary to tinker with players and systems to get the team to GEL together – once this is up and running over a period of time, and the coach is satisfied: it should be left alone.

Tinkering with the team players should only be done for a genuine reason – for example, if there are injuries to some players, not fully fit or not playing well. Tinkering with the system of play for no genuine reason can also cause problems for the coach, and team. Tinkering with players is bad enough - tinkering with the system and players at the same time, makes it even more difficult to assess problems when things go wrong.

This is the coach's responsibility, and it is his / her call – but it is advisable to stick to the team, and system that is performing with optimum efficiency – week in week out. It is the coach's responsibility to play his strongest team for any competitive game regardless of the venue or level of competition – he / she owe this to themselves, the players, and the fans. The coach or manager must make this a STATUTORY rule - and only make changes when some players are not performing to the optimum standard required – or forced on by injured players unable to play.
When a coach or manager does not play his strongest team, it reduces the team's standard of play, and this gives the opponent a mental and physical boost: and most times they raise the standard of their game to make it very difficult for the coach or manager and team. Playing your strongest team increases confidence – consistency and continuity amongst the team. Do not make wholesale changes to the team, if changes are to be made: it should be done with a certain amount of subtlety and not interfere with the team's performance.

Remember - if it's not broken do not fix it.

Making substitutions at the right time is not an easy option at the best of times. Substitution should not be made for the sake of it, there should be a reason for doing so: one common mistake a coach or manager tend to make is to take off one or two of the best players, especially when they are playing well, and replace them with players of lesser quality - this can cause the team to become incoherent, and can lose the game. Substitution of this kind is not a good idea, and should not be repeated. Protect the players from hidden dangers – sidetrack. The coach or manager can only do so much – players will have to help themselves – a team effort in any language.

The basic mental picture of the game should be the same for coach and players: the coach and players should read the manual to bring their mental pictures together to be on the same wavelength as each other.

Sometimes, circumstances beyond the control of the coach, and players occur and this affects the team's performance. It is not easy, but the coach and players will have to rise above it - regroup and reassert themselves.
Making sure, the players do not abuse their life styles, by over indulging in alcohol, drug or other destructive sidelines – not an easy problem – how do you protect a man from himself or a woman from herself - the coach, cannot watch a player 24 hours a day, and the player will need to have some self - discipline to help himself or herself for a certain amount of self control for their BEHAVIOUR on and off the pitch.
A footballer no matter good he or she is, who lacks discipline should be nipped in the bud, and if he or she does not respond positively, then there is the door: this is one of many of the coach's responsibilities.
The coach / manager should not enforce his / her limitation upon player's aspirations for no reason. The coach / manager, and players should not let fame or fortune go to their heads and must behave responsibly.
The coach / manager should not tolerate players who are persistent troublemakers: on the other hand, the coach / manager should be firm, but fair and gradually harmony and respect will develop on both sides.
If a player is unhappy, and wants to leave for some reason the manager should let that player go.
The coach should make sure that his / her players can defend, and attack for ninety minutes plus extra time, and to keep the game flowing: players must not stop, and wait for a linesman to flag or a referee to blow his / her whistle for a decision: this produces a break in the game, and gives the opponent a chance to gain possession, and a possibility to score.

The coach or manager should clock the players, and this includes the goalkeeper for the time to run various distances in acceptable times, in both training and playing; the times should be approximately the same in both instances. The runs of the players should be done with and without the ball in a straight line motion, and also, the coach or manager, should take note to see, if, the players are applying Newton's first law of motion when changing the direction of a run with the ball – to enhance complete control of player and ball.
Do not try to go beyond your velocity, and acceleration limit: the coach or manager in conjunction with the players should work out the optimum limit of each player. Because every player is different, in build, stamina, and strength, energy levels, etc., players should not be forced to do something that he / she cannot do or what is wrong or dangerous to do. The coach / manager should employ a trained high jump specialist teacher to teach the players how to leap and land safely when heading a ball in defence or attack to an optimum standard. The coach or manager should make sure the team players concentrate, and be focused on the task in hand and not lose the game.
When a coach or manager is employed to manage a football club – he / she, and only he / she should have the responsibilities of running the club: he / she should be in charge of training – picking the team – buying and selling players: assisting coaching staffs will also have their responsibilities, and they must keep in touch with the coach or manager. If the coach or manager so wishes he /she may employ an engineer, or technical analyst with a fluid and particle dynamics discipline, and football / soccer knowledge: to advise him / her on any engineering or technical aspects of play; if certain departments of play needs to be improved, whenever some technical problems arises or needs clarification. This advisory position will, also be under the control of the coach or manager.
The coach, players, and advisor must think as one unit. There must be no interference from anyone else – except if, and when the team is performing very badly and is reflected in a low position in the table – and there are no signs of improvement – only then, the chairman / directors should intervene and find better coaching staffs - but they should be given more than enough time to get things up and running.

Sending Off Players by the Referee

The referee will send players off, if he / she find them persistently breaking the football / soccer rules. Players must think of the consequences of being sent off. This causes many problems for the coach / manager, and the team – especially, if a player or players are sent off early in the game. The coach / /manager has to reshuffle his original plan, and players have to work even harder to compensate for the loss of players sent off. The remaining players have to expend a lot more energy to keep the high standard of play that is required to keep the game flowing and to avoid defeat. So players must try very hard to avoid breaking the football / soccer rules during the ninety minutes, plus extra time of play.

Fighting By Players - On and Off the Pitch

Intended head butting and fists fights on the pitch during the game must be avoided. If a team-mate is involved in a potentially explosive situation, another team-mate must react and respond quickly to diffuse and pull away his / her team-mate out of trouble: this applies to off the pitch as well.
This type of behaviour has a bad affect on the game – it disrupts the flow of the game – players could be yellow or red carded – players tend to lose concentration and focus – and this sets a bad example for youngsters to copy. It does not make sense, and it's not worth it.
Players must learn to walk away from this type of situation – because when you have calmed down, you will see that you have made the right decision: remember it is harder to walk away.
Volatile energy is best channelled into playing good football, and not to get involved in any silly ideas.

Verbal Abuse - All Types - From Opposing Fans

This is an inflammatory subject, and stems from a minority within the crowd who likes to wind up the opponents. Sometimes these people do not know when to stop or where to draw the line. This type of conduct is no good for football, because football is for everybody to enjoy.
The coach / manager or players are in a position to do very little to combat it – but the football authorities at all levels can, and should ban the teams or countries for a number of games, and points deducted, if they do not sort out the problems. In this way this type of behaviour by some of these people will improve, and eventually be stamped out.
When goals are scored, celebrations by some players should be kept to a minimum, and the players be focused for the re-start of play. This is a critical time for the team's reaction and response to be at its best, because this is a time where the opponent can strike back quickly to score.
If the coach or manager so desires, he / she may use the PVT relationship to change things around to help the team to perform better, in attack or defence or both, as he / she see fit at any point in time during the game.
Whichever style the coach chooses to play by stick to that style and get better and better with it. If you decide to change the style to another one, you can do so, but get better and better with it.
When things go wrong – ask deep searching questions – assess the situation, and find solutions to the problems, most of which are in this manual, some are physically visible and others are mentally hidden: in either or both cases, will have to be assessed, and solutions found.
There are two types of coach/manager –the good and the bad. The good coach/manager is one who is humble, and willing to learn, adapt to new and better ideas, and implement them for the better of the team and football-soccer with a high level of success.
The bad coach/manager is one who has a bad attitude, is not humble, not willing to learn, not willing to adapt to new and better ideas, and in some ways, has an illusion of "know it all" "seen it all" "done it all" who almost always gets the sack or jumps from one club to another with little or no success.

Chapter 3

Analogies – Cliché and Terms

The analogies – cliché and terms given in this manual, are to show how they are related to football – soccer managers, and players. Implementing these under various circumstances will help the coach, manager, and players to maintain the very high standard required by this manual.

Two words to help you remember after learning - these are INTEREST and CONCENTRATION.
Learn and remember the following –

1. The truth is the only correct answer.
2. Football is not about who is right – but what is right – do what is right – get it right – keep it right. Sometimes, if you are anxious to do what is right; you forget to do what is right; so you have to be careful with your thoughts – when a choice has to be made between two rights use priority.
3. How do you fight an idea? You fight an idea with a better idea – and a better idea is: Practice makes perfect: but Perfect Practice makes perfect is a better idea, and forms the basis of this system. Perfect Practice has limitations, and precautions must be taken, in order that injury can be avoided or kept to a minimum by the players. It will be impossible to achieve 100 % Perfect Practice because of our human nature, but if you can achieve 90 – 95 % you will have gone a long way to achieving your goal.
4. Choosing a way to loose – what's the difference? Choosing a way to win that's the hard part - stick with the hard part: and the hard part is mental and physical Perfect Practices that the players should practice during training and playing on match days to get right.
5. Football is like acting, where Perfectly Practice thoughts are transformed into Perfectly Practice play: here the manual is the script, the coach is the director and the players are the actors: bring them together and they produce a game of breathtaking displays.
6. Patience is one of the hardest things to achieve, because it is the one thing that is always working against your nature.
7. The river analogy: football is like a river – always takes the path of least resistance, and has the following properties: beautiful – turbulent – kinetic and potential energy – streamline – width – depth – attack – defence – widens – narrows – weaves – twist and turn – calm, change of pace – deceptive – interchanges, inter–passes, always creating an opening – always going forward.
8. The "QUEEN HORNET" and "QUEEN BEE" ANALOGY for defence. When the hornets, and bees protect their queen – they do so quickly, fearlessly, and to the end: the hornets, and bees seek out and close down the opponents, and so, in a football / soccer game defenders must follow the hornets, and bees natural instinct to protect their goalkeeper, and goal area to get in FRONT of the opponents, and nearest to the ball – two or three defending team-mates to surround the opponent, and fairly take the ball away from him / her – to get rid of the ball from dangerous areas or start a move, as quickly, and safely as possible: whenever their goal is threatened. The hornet and bee workers are PROMPTED by their natural instinct to defend, and protect their hives to the very end.
9. Equal weight pull – stranded cable wire. When some of the wires in a support cable, are badly stranded – the cable will not be able to withstand the load it was intended for. If a load is applied to the cable, some of the individual wires that are properly stranded will support the load, and the badly stranded wires will not. As the load is increased the good stranded wires becomes weaker, and eventually breaks: because of the extra work load taken up by the good stranded wires, and the badly stranded wires supporting little or no load. Some wires are working hard, and some are not. The whole cable is not functioning 100% - this is like a football team, where some players pull their weight, and some do not. Unequal weight pull causes continuous separation of some players in the team, and prevents the team from functioning as one unit. It is vital that all team players pull their weight equally during the 90 minutes plus extra time of play.
10. Hidden dangers to coach and players. Side–track: The powerful hidden danger which overrides the emotion and minds: reduces their power of concentration and ability to focus 100% on football.

Instead of the coach or players, focusing on their Perfect Practices in training to play good football – remembering what they supposed to do on a match day: the coach or players or both end up with no ideas or very little to offer on match days. Mental sabotage characterised by hostile or friendly propaganda: opponent attempts to wear down or build-up players / coaches, by the gradual division – destruction of harmony, and morale within the team and other personnel. Unsettling media cover, this is a ploy hatched up by opponents in different ways, for example, good or bad, media cover, reports, interviews, to disrupt the coach or players powers of concentration – generally putting them off their game plan. A bad ploy could make you angry: a good ploy could make you elated; they are effective and usually produce bad results called divide and conquer. In addition, the coach and players must be in control of the following hidden dangers - complacency – arrogance – ball watching – anger – temper – revenge – blames – argument – and over celebrating a goal - do not fall in the TRAP and do not fall at the last fence.

11. First you play with your heads, and then with your hearts.
12. The three "Cs" – confidence – consistency and continuity.
13. The three "Ds" – desire – devotion – and discipline.
14. The three "Ss" – strength – stamina and speed.
15. If the opponent cannot score: the opponent cannot win - A CLEAN SHEET. If you score more goals than the opponent – the opponent cannot win. In a sword fight – the person who loses his / her sword usually loses the fight. If a player loses the ball: he / she could lose the game.
16. Prevention is better than cure – the team that makes the least amount of mistakes will win the game.
17. Strength in numbers.
18. Fear makes you go backwards: get your mental and physical Perfect Practices right – keep it right and this will help you to conquer fear and go forward.
19. Power is no good without precision, useful for the defining moment of the final ball.
20. Pressure – force per unit area: when a wall is to be knocked down, a certain amount of force has to be applied: when enough force is applied, the wall starts to crack at its weakest point – application of more pressure, and the wall starts to fall apart. Pressure must be applied to the opponents to force them back: cause them to become edgy – make all sorts of errors in defence: and eventually fall apart. Relentless pressure is the best type of pressure to apply to the opponents – critical times.
21. The slow process – this is where the standard, in one or more departments of play, has fallen too low without the coach / manager or players realising it – it's like a car getting old - reflected in increasing poor performance: high standard must be maintained at all times.
22. For every action: there is a reaction – Newton's third law of motion.
23. Regardless of the competition, the venue might be different, but the reasons for playing to win are the same – remember the hard part – Perfect Practice.
24. First, fast and in front of the opponent.
25. The team that wants it most is the team that wins.
26. Greediness and foolishness – a lethal combination: think and avoid.
27. Cool – composed – a calm head with self – determination.
28. Scoring goals is a serious business, but it should also be fun.
29. Play to win, you may get a win or a draw: play for a draw, you may get a draw, but almost always you will lose.
30. Do not sit back on a lead – consolidate lead and position.
31. Players must stop only, when the referee blows his/ her whistle during the game – at half time interval – and at full time. Players must not stop during the game, and hope the referee will blow the whistle for whatever reason they have stopped for. This gives chances to the opponent, and must be avoided.
32. The dynamics of football – soccer, is the relationship between the forces of nature, players and ball.
33. Four words that could help you through life and football – soccer: "watch your back jack".
34. In football / soccer - one team is going somewhere, the other is going nowhere.

35. Trust – this is a difficult situation or risky business, because at times you have to trust someone: but the safest option is to trust no one: then they cannot betray you – it's your call.
36. When you talk about how you are going to implement your mental and physical Perfect Practice – just don't talk about; go out and do it.
37. If the opponent does not have the ball – the opponent cannot play, so don't give the ball away.
38. If it is not broken – do not fix it; that is, if the team is playing well leave it alone – the coach or manager should not tinker with the team or make wholesale changes to suit any situation. The same team should be kept together for as long as possible to get better and better: also if there is a second team or a reserve team – this team should also be playing to the optimum standard of the first team, so if the coach or manager is forced to make a change with one or two players from the second team to the first team, these players will be able to fit into the first team as if there were no changes made: making sure the Perfect Practice is carried out on the training ground prior to the game.
39. If you allow hate, anger and retribution to get the upper hand – they will put your timing out - THINK before you say or do anything: or before you do something, think of how you are going to do it, before you do it.
40. Do what you do, as long as it is right: and do it well.
41. Ask not of what football can do for the manager and players, but what the manager and players can do for football.
42. If you make £100.00 per week for example, save half of it, and live on just the other half.
43. Split loyalty – sometimes you have to make a choice or torn between two or more things etc., think and do what is right - use priority, firmness, and fairness.
44. A drawn game is better than a lost game, one point is better than no point, and a small fish is better than an empty dish.
45. Perfect Practices on the training ground and on match days with humility, quiet optimism.

.

46. Cruelty stems from misery – avoid.
47. Do not allow your stupidity to override your ability – avoid.
48. Do not take anything or anyone for granted whilst enjoying the benefits of modern civilization.
49. Knowledge is power – put it to good use.
50. Do not spend more money than you make - for if you do, you will enter trouble times, this applies to owners, clubs, coaches/managers, and players.

Chapter 4

Team Players - optimum ages 17yrs to 27yrs

The Goalkeeper – is an integral part of defence – all players to avoid head injuries in set-play.

The goalkeeper should have the following qualities – he / she should be tall, brave, and fit. He / she should, also be mentally strong, smart and decisive – able to resist intimidation from opponents – good eyesight: keep eyes on the ball – ability to jump high and collect crosses: cleanly – or to punch clear – to dive low get down quickly and spread himself / herself to stop ball. Narrowing angles – be in the right position at the right time: move quickly, from one side of the goal to the other, to stop the ball from going in.

An accurate kicker and thrower of the ball especially to a team-mate to team-mate for passing.
Good stopper of short and long-range power drives – always alert.
Do not get caught napping during play.
Work closely with his / her defenders: keep them on their toes.
Direct his / her defenders in building a wall when free kicks are to be taken in and around dangerous areas making it difficult for the kicker to score: deny the opponent space.
Shouts should be loud, clear, and decisive.
Watch for and get defenders to close down UNMARKED OPPONENTS in dangerous 18 yd / penalty area during the game when defending, set pieces, corners, long throws – and free kicks.
Do not allow any FREE HEADERS by an opponent.
The goalkeeper should not give the ball away to the opponent by way of a bad pass; kick – throw or allow the ball to bounce off carelessly to the opponent – understand Newton's first law for better ball control p.50.
When a ball is struck fiercely to the keeper – he / she must be able to deal with it in a positive way – plenty of Perfect Practice needs to be carried out by the goalkeeper: to learn to cushion the ball at the moment of contact: to reduce the impact, momentum and kinetic energy of the ball, without losing the ball, giving the ball to the opponent or allowing the ball to get into the net. Some shots may be too hard to hold on to: in this case, the keeper must punch clear with both fists away to safety, and away from the opponent: tip over the bar or turn around the posts – a decision the goal keeper has to make, at that point of time. In addition to the Perfect Practice the goalkeeper must do – is to get his / her fitness level to a high standard in the department of short burst of velocity, and acceleration between the goalposts, and within his / her 18 yd / penalty area. The faster he / she accelerate and dive towards the turf or get down quickly or accelerate and leap upwards: the better it is for him / her to get the ball first. This needs Perfect Practice for velocity against time of the ball struck by the opponent. The goalkeeper is the only member of the team who is allowed to touch or hold the ball with his / her hands in the 18yd/penalty area, and ROLL it out to a team-mate for tight passing.

THE GOALKEEPER'S LINE

The goalkeeper must be decisive in his/her choice of – know when to stay on his / her line or when to come out, he / she must not be caught in no man's land: here quick thinking – reaction and response with respect to time, velocity, and distance of keeper and ball, are the required factors. The goal line is the BASE for the keeper to work from.

The goalkeeper off his /her line has a greater distance to cover in order to tip the ball over the bar, punch clear or collect the ball coming in under the bar. This is an important factor which the goalkeeper must keep in mind, is his / her position with respect to the goal line, Fig. 1 – 4.
If an opponent takes a free kick just outside the 18 yd box defended by a wall, and if, the ball rises over the wall, and starts to dip under the bar: the goalkeeper should be in a position, to tip the ball over the bar, punch clear or collect the ball. The goalkeeper can only do so, if he / she is on the goal line because the goalkeeper has to cover less distance to reach the ball.

Now if, the goalkeeper is, say for example 3 or 4 metres off the goal line, Fig. 2 – 4 and the ball is coming in and starts to dip under the bar – the goalkeeper will have to run backwards to try and get to the ball: by this time the ball would have gone under the bar, because the goalkeeper had to cover 3 or 4 metres before leaping to get the ball – the goalkeeper is selling himself / herself short of TIME and SPACE.
It is easier for the goalkeeper to run or accelerate in a forward direction than it is in a backward direction. If the ball happens to fall short off the goalkeeper's line, he / she has a good chance to wait for the ball or get to the ball, because he / she can run or accelerate in a forward direction quicker than in backward direction, plus the keeper can control the ball better going forward than going backward – he / she can have more control of the body's centre of gravity to help control the ball.

Goalkeeper on His / Her Line

Fig. 1 – 4 the goalkeeper is on his / her line, and is able to tip the ball over the bar.

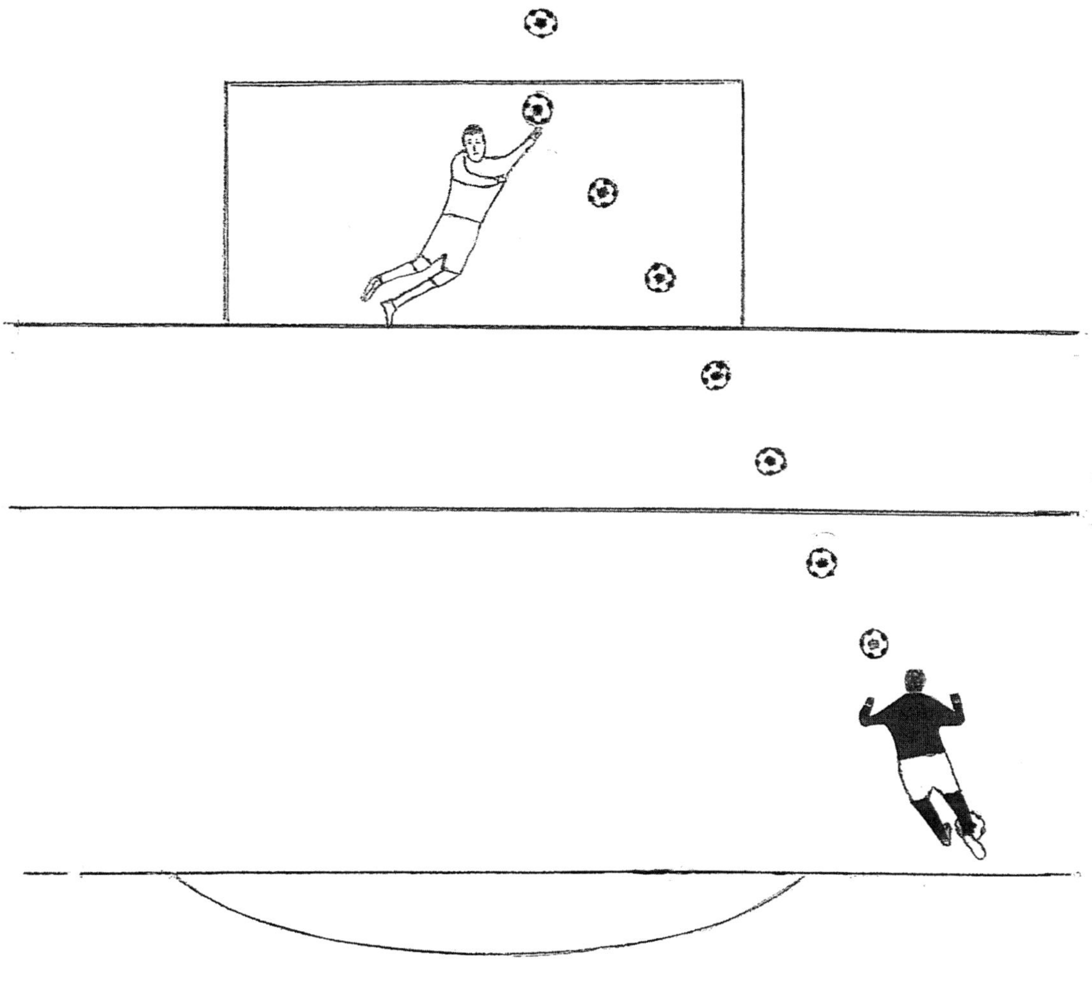

Goalkeeper off His / Her Line

Fig. 2 – 4 the goalkeeper is off his / her line, and is unable to get to the ball which enters the net.

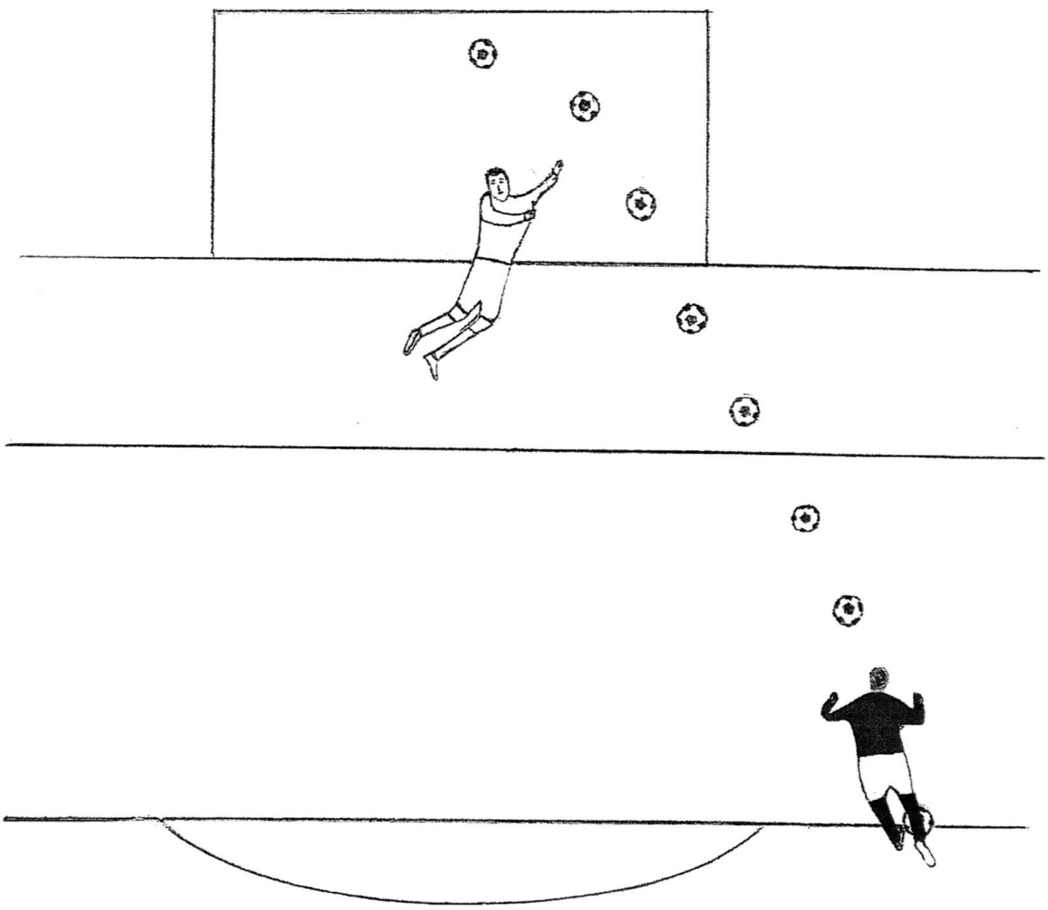

The goalkeeper must try to throw or roll the ball out to his team-mates, his / her back 3 / 4 or midfield players to start a move and to keep possession. The goalkeeper should not try to kick a ball that is moving towards his / her goal mouth – unless circumstances forces him / her to do so: he / she must get their bodies behind the ball, use the hands to cushion and hold on to the ball – tip over the bar or punch clear.

The goalkeeper, when in a "one on one" situation with the opponent striker will have to keep the legs close together in order to increase the blocking surface area to stop the ball from going through the legs – and into the net – try to be in a position to either leap or dive with his / her body behind the ball.

One Bounce Ball – with forward or backward spin - good reaction and response

To deal with the one bounce ball, Fig. 3 – 4 the goalkeeper makes a good judgement, for the increase in velocity of the ball caused by the bounce, and spin to get his /her body behind the ball, and cushion it to absorb the extra kinetic energy gained by the ball due to the bounce, spin, and slide. If the goalkeeper thinks he / she cannot hold on to the ball then the goalkeeper must decisively punch clear to safety.

One Bounce Ball – with forward or backward spin - bad reaction and response

In Fig. 4 – 4, the keeper makes a bad judgment for the increase in velocity of the ball – caused by the bounce, and spin is unable to get his / her body behind the ball before it goes past into the net. (See ball motion in Chapter 5). The keeper must avoid this and not allow it to happen.

On The Turf Ball – good reaction and response

When the ball is coming on the turf towards the keeper Fig. 5 - 4 he / she gets down quickly – get his / her body on the turf and behind the ball; and hold on to it – there must be no gaps between the keeper's body and the turf for the ball to pass through – good timing of the keeper moving downwards in relation to the ball coming towards the keeper are essential in getting the body behind the ball – good reaction and equally good response is needed to deal with this situation.

On The Turf Ball – bad reaction and response

Fig. 6 – 4 shows the keeper gets his / her timing wrong – the keeper's reaction and response is slow, and is unable to get his / her body behind the ball, and the ball goes through the gap and into the net – the keeper must avoid this and not allow it to happen.

One Bounce Ball – good reaction and response

Fig. 3 – 4 the goalkeeper makes a good reaction and response to get his / her body behind the ball, and was prepared for the change in velocity of the ball – caused by the bounce of the ball.

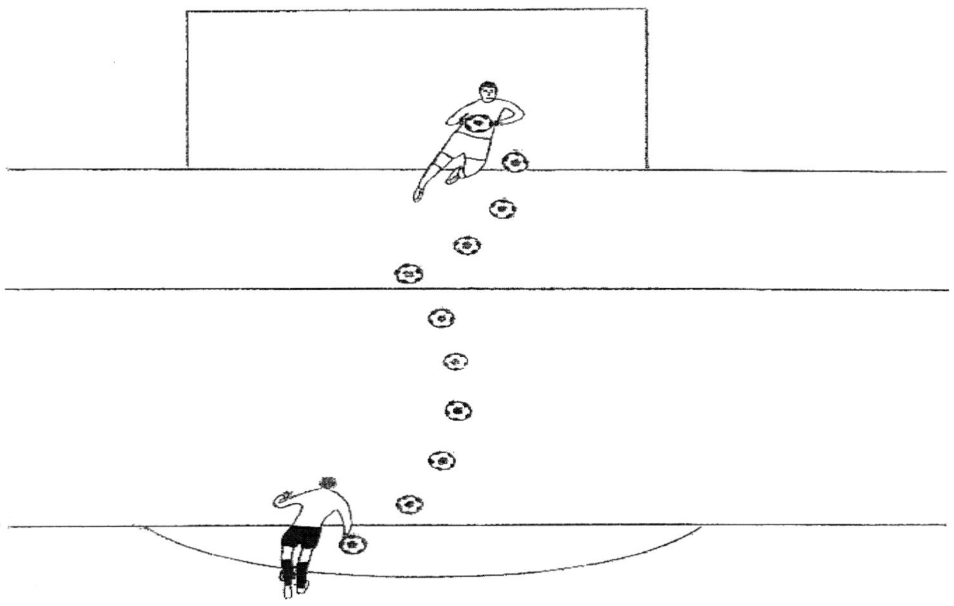

One Bounce Ball – bad reaction and response

Fig. 4 – 4 the goalkeeper is caught flat–footed because he / she did not allow for the bounce, and increase in velocity of the ball – the goalkeeper's reaction and response to get his / her body behind the ball is slow – keeper misses the ball before it enters the net.

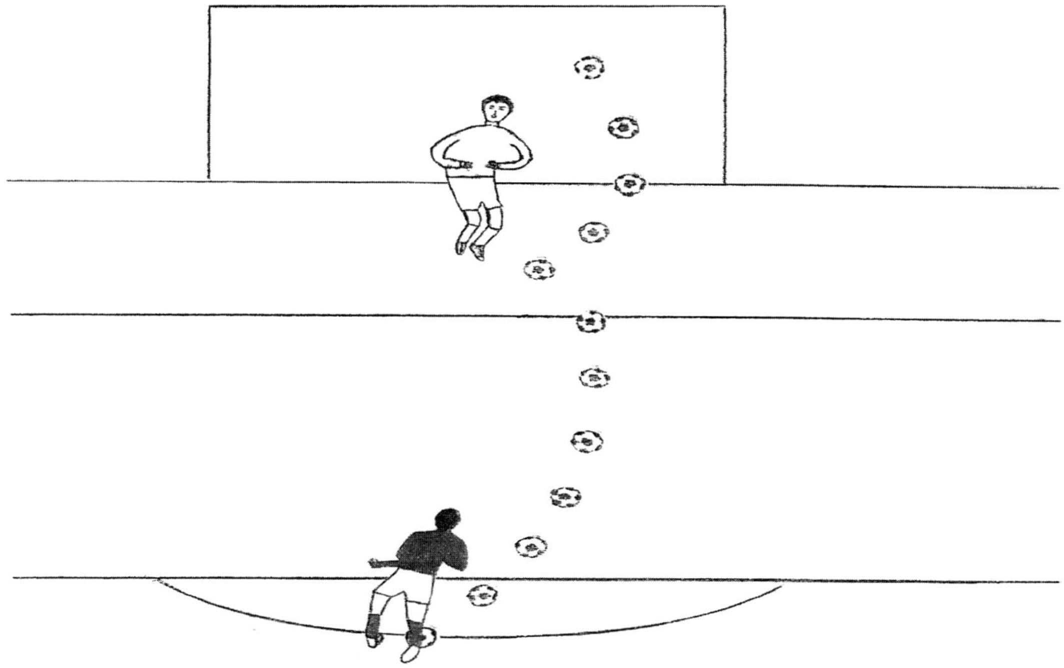

On The Turf Ball – good timing

Fig. 5 – 4 the goalkeeper makes a quick reaction and response to get his / her body behind the ball – keeper's timing and downward velocity to the turf, with respect to the velocity of the incoming ball is good.

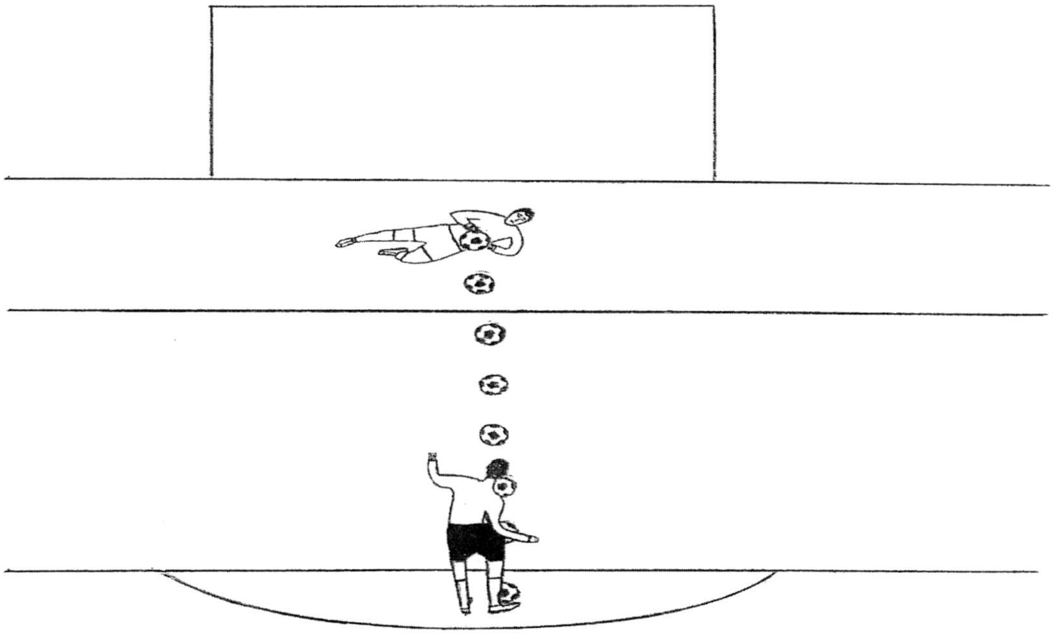

On The Turf Ball – bad timing

Fig. 6 – 4 the goalkeeper makes a slow reaction and response, and is unable to get his / her body behind the ball – keeper's timing and downward velocity to turf, with respect to the velocity of the incoming ball is bad.

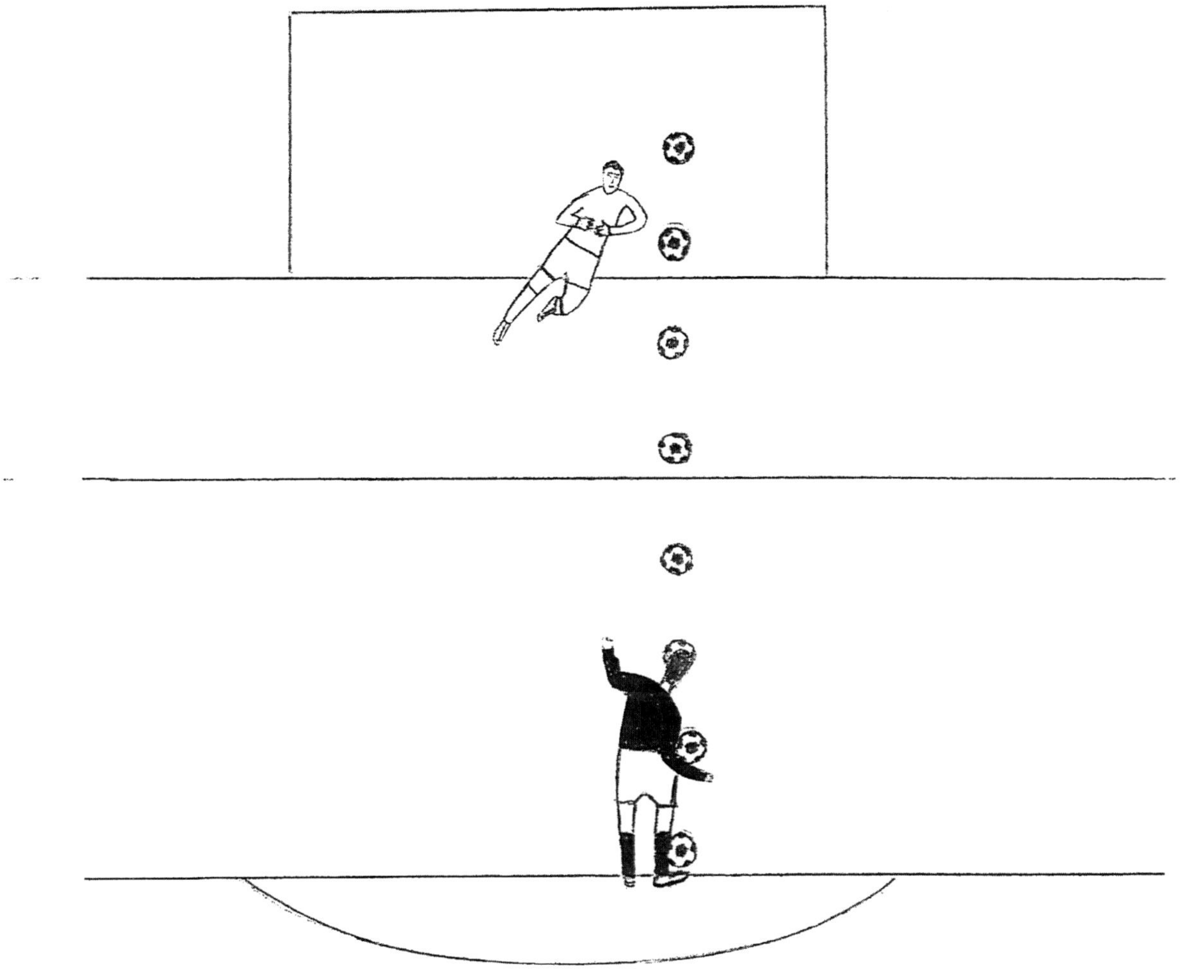

The Right and Left Backs

The right and left backs are players of similar qualities, to those of the centre backs, except for the positions in which they play: the right and left side of the pitch.
Must be mentally alert during the game, good co-ordination and understanding with centre backs, goalkeeper, midfield players, and strikers, do not go to sleep, during the game.
A firm well timed tackler – one who goes for the ball – a ball winner. One who looks up, before making slide rule crosses or passes to an UNMARKED team-mate.
Quick – early close down, shields the ball from opponents.
No hesitation head and feet clearances must be made.
Good in the air and a very tight marker of the opponent.
Able to defend and attack in a split second: quick reaction and response time.
Organise defence – watch out and close down UNMARKED OPPONENTS – ESPECIALLY SET PIECES- NO FREE HEADERS by opponents.
Stay in position to defend and protect the goalkeeper – and goal area – defend his/her area for 90 minutes plus extra time. When the right back goes up or goes forward to link up with the midfield or strikers: the remaining back 3 /4 must stay in position to counteract any quick breaks from the opponents. Do not leave the back door wide open, because of surprise over the top or through balls by the opponent.
Do not give the opponents, TIME and COMPLETE space.
Possess dynamic qualities, such as good velocity, acceleration, and retardation – sudden change of pace – sudden change of direction and to understand Newton's first law of motion for better ball control. Perfect – Practice how to produce the DEFINING MOMENT IN DEFENCE and the DEFINING MOMENT OF THE FINAL BALL.

Centre Backs

The centre backs should be tall, strong and commanding. Good in the air, and good with both feet: ability to control, and dictates the game from the back to spread the play. Able to hold on to the ball – hold off opponents – shield the ball, and look up, before making that vital slide rule cross or pass to his / her team – mate in TOTAL ISOLATION.
Good co-ordination, and understanding, with the right back, left back, goalkeeper, midfield players, and strikers.
The pillars in defence - firm, but fair tacklers, and winners of the ball.
They must attack incoming corners with precision.
Should be the CAPTAIN, to keep team-mates under control, focused and well organised. Reads the game – anticipate opponents – intercept crosses and passes from opponents.
Watch out for and mark tightly the UNMARKED OPPONENTS in dangerous areas - getting in FRONT of the opponents at all times.
Good intelligent back–tracking, after going forward. Does not give the opponents TIME and COMPLETE SPACE: always in the right place at the right time.
Possess dynamic qualities such as good velocity, acceleration, retardation, sudden change of pace, and direction and to understand Newton's first law of motion for better ball control.
Play for 90 minutes plus extra time. Perfect Practice how to produce - the DEFINING MOMENT IN DEFENCE - and the DEFINING MOMENT OF THE FINAL BALL.

Midfield Players

Midfield players – right, central and left sides should be strong, fast and with stamina to play for 90 minutes plus extra time; defend and attack.

Good co-ordination – and understanding with goalkeeper, the back 3 / 4 and strikers. Beware of ball watching during the game.
Every player must pull their weight equally: and do not give the opponent TIME and COMPLETE SPACE – safe head and feet clearances when necessary.
Link up with back 3 / 4 or forward as they see fit.
Break down early build-up by opponents, with good anticipation – quick reaction time, and sharp closing down of opponents.
Intercept opponent passes – look for and close down UNMARKED OPPONENTS. Close down opponents before they can put their passes together – deny them the ball.

Look up before making slide rule passes to an UNMARKED team-mate.
Possession is the key – keeping the ball – making strings of UNBROKEN slide rule crosses and passes to team-mates: right down to the final ball. If you lose the ball – win it back quickly.
Score long-range goals 25yd/m when linking up with forwards.

Midfield HOLDING players – these are players who holds their midfield positions – while other midfield players goes forward in attack; for example, two goes up: two stays back to control the midfield areas.
Possess dynamic qualities such as, good velocity, acceleration and retardation, change of direction, and to use Newton's first law of motion for better ball control. Perfect practice THE DEFINING MOMENT IN DEFENCE and THE DEFINING MOMENT OF THE FINAL BALL.

Right and Left Wingers – are the fuel supply lines

Similar type of flank players, some likes the right, some likes the left, and some don't mind which side they play on. Quick, strong with close ball control good footwork, very tricky with step-over.
Good co-ordination, and understanding with team-mates during the game – run down the flank, dribbling, going past defenders – looking up before crossing or passing the ball across the face of the opponent goal: or making varied angled cut backs to the UNMARKED team-mate waiting or moving away from their marker in the opponent 18 yd / penalty area.
Put strings of UNBROKEN slide rule crosses and passes together – right down to the final ball – to interchange – inter-pass – exchange passes with team-mates in the opponent 18 yd / penalty area – to the unmarked team–mate in SPLENDID ISOLATION.
The winger can also go it alone and score with the keeper unaware: the element of surprise attack.
Good defender and attacker – do not ball watch when team-mates are struggling to win the ball: get in there, and help dispossess the opponent, without getting in each other's way.
Possess dynamic qualities such as, good velocity – acceleration – and retardation – sudden change of pace – sudden change of direction and to understand Newton's first law for better ball control.

The "Hold Up" Player – a striker, winger or midfield player who can get in the opponent 18 yd / penalty area – a player who can zigzag dribble with step-over – twist and turn – send opponents the wrong way – shield the ball – keep possession – lay off passes – set up chances, and half chances to the UNMARKED team-mates deep in the opponent 18 yd / penalty area, teases the opponent and keeper before scoring – a naturally gifted tricky player, with good footwork – cool – calm and composed with mesmerising skills.
When the winger runs with the ball, and has an opponent in pursuit trying to close him / her down – the winger has the problem of fending off the opponent, like riding tackles to keep possession - that is, the winger's acceleration, velocity, and the inertia he / she gives the ball must be correct, he / she must not over-hit or under-hit the ball. If the winger decides to put the ball across the face of the opponent goal as he / she runs down the flank, at some point the winger will have to reduce his / her velocity and change direction

of the ball to get a slide rule pass across the face of goal. The winger's run in this case is related to Newton's first law of motion: if the winger does not slow down before he / she changes direction to strike the ball across the face of goal, the player will tend to maintain the velocity and direction he / she originally possessed which means that the ball will be sent in another direction or off target instead of being square or parallel to the face of goal. Perfect Practice - how to produce the DEFINING MOMENT IN DEFENCE AND THE DEFINING MOMENT OF THE FINAL BALL.

Centre Forward

This player is most comfortable in the opponent 18 yd / penalty area.
Player must be good in the air – and also good with both feet.
Quick – strong and clinical finisher. Ability to control and hold on to crosses and passes from wingers and other team-mates. Good defender, with ability to dispossess the opponent and keep the ball – run at defenders, dummy, twist turn and dribble past opponents on his way to score. Look up – make slide rule crosses and passes to an UNMARKED team-mate – become a provider sometimes, and score goals at other times, depending on who is in the best goal scoring position – snap up half chances.
Ability to inter-pass, interchange and exchange UNBROKEN crosses and passes with UNMARKED team - mates in the opponent 18 yd / penalty area.
Beat opponent keeper; with "one on one" run, know exactly how to get past the keeper by way of chips – dummy – swerve – go around keeper – or put ball through keeper's leg.
Must not ball watch during the game: if, you see the opponent with the ball: get in there and dispossess the opponent – keep possession. Make safe, decisive head and feet clearances when the opponents are in dangerous areas.
Possess dynamic qualities such as, good velocity – acceleration – and retardation – sudden change of pace – sudden change of direction and to understand Newton's first law of motion for better ball control. Perfect Practice - how to produce the DEFINING MOMENT IN DEFENCE and THE DEFINING MOMENT OF THE FINAL BALL.
THE "FASTEST DRIBBLER" – any team player who could clock 100 metres in 10 seconds or under, and run/dribble with the ball at his / her feet at the same time to set up chances for his / her team-mates to score.

Formations

The coach / manager may use any formation to play from. The key is to use TWO WINGERS with the chosen formation. It is important to stick to the formation – especially in defence: so the goalkeeper, and back 3 /4 know exactly, where each player is – in relation to their positions. This keeps co-ordination and understanding between players up to its high standard.

During the run of play, the formation is constantly changing – so it as important, that the last line of defence, the back 3 / 4 does not get caught out of position with the goalkeeper on his own.

Some common formations normally used are -

4	3	3
4	4	2
3	4	3

The 3 2 5 formation with one inside right and one inside left players linking back and forth, with the midfield, strikers and defence – depending on the possession – and when support is needed in defence or attack. So, in effect it's a 3 2 5 becoming a 3 4 3 and vice-versa during the game – a very exciting formation, which produces the element of surprise to the opponent with plenty of fire power up front.

Perfect Practice

The Horizontal and Vertical Planes

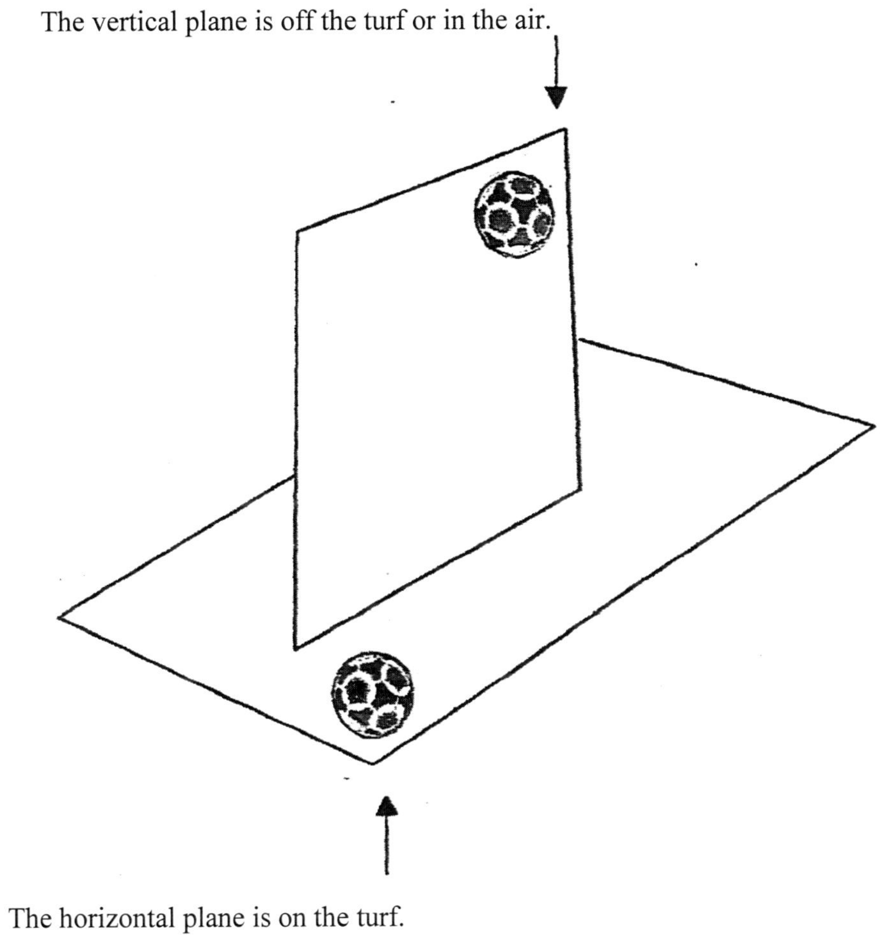

Fig. 7 – 4

Some teams can defend and attack in the horizontal plane – some teams can defend and attack in the vertical plane – but good teams defend and attack in both the horizontal and vertical planes.

Pitch Dimensions

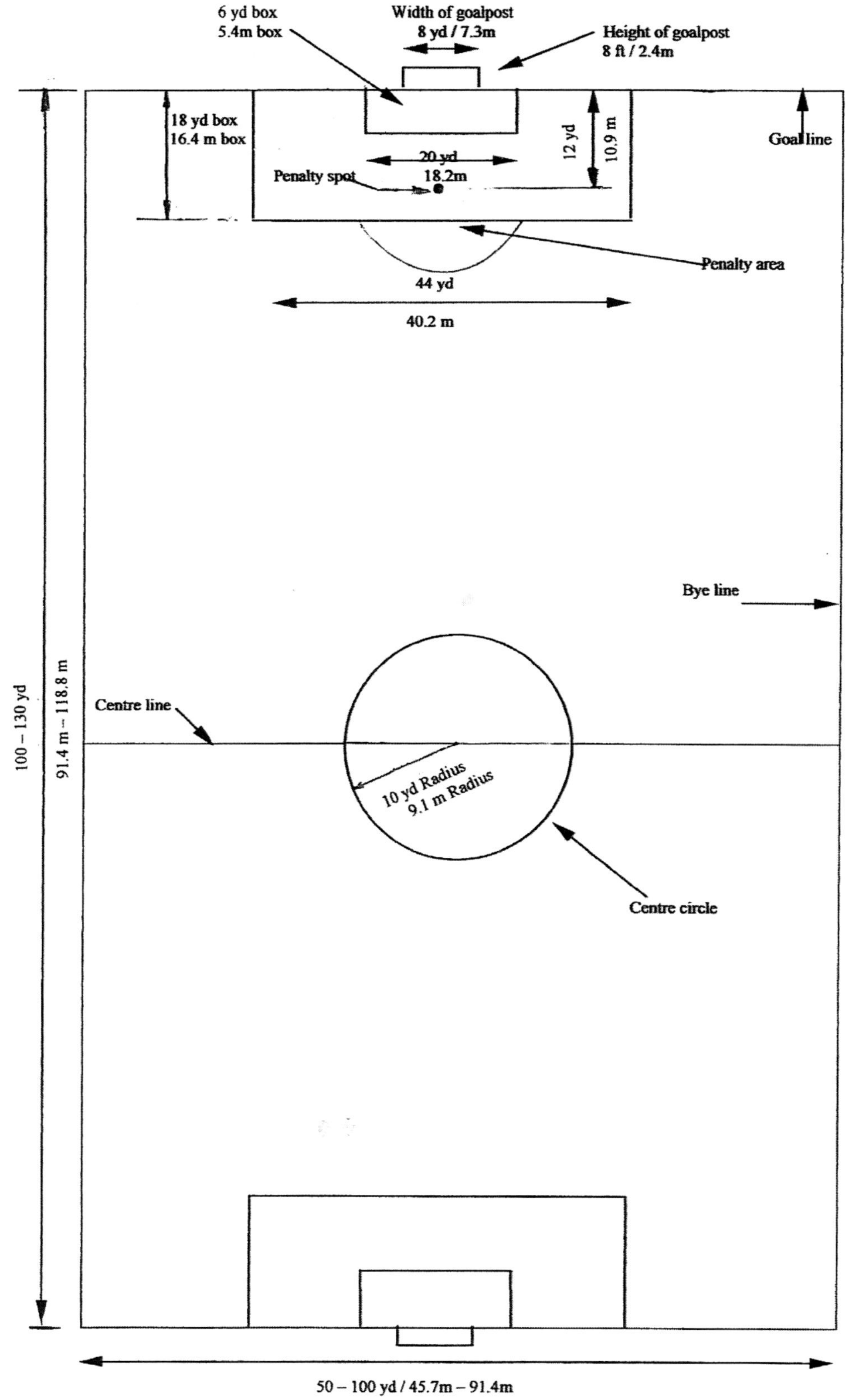

Fig. 8 – 4

Chapter 5

Basic Fluid and Particle Dynamics

Concepts of Fluid Flow - River System and Ball Dynamics

The object of this Chapter is to show the similarity between a free flowing river- fluid and that of free flowing football- soccer. How the forces of nature affect the problems to be analysed in both cases: how to apply the basic principles of fluid and particle dynamics to arrive at suitable analytical solutions – and how to react and respond to various fluid and particle dynamics situations, as they arise during training and playing – for example, the importance of velocity and acceleration of the player with respect to other team-mates – the ball – distances and time in closing down an opponent, to get the ball first or to find out why the ball did not hit the target: and when to use Newton's first law of motion, absorb or divert kinetic energy etc,.

Some problems in fluid and particle dynamics can be solved using basic mathematics; others require the application of elementary or advanced calculus. For the purpose of this manual basic mathematics are used, and it is assumed that most players will have attained an ordinary level of mathematics: but do not worry if you have not; you can play good football with a little knowledge, natural ability and common sense.

Fluid and particle dynamics are used in many branches of science, and engineering – to sports in general and to football / soccer in particular. Today's fluid and particle dynamics are the result of great work done by scientists and engineers such as Newton – Reynolds – Bernoulli – Magnus, and Prandtl.

Concepts of fluid flow

Fluid is defined as a substance that takes the shape of the containing vessel. Fluid flow is complex – due to different types of flows with varying velocities, and accelerations. There are three important concepts of fluid flow, and these are – the principle of mass; kinetic energy and momentum. Fluid flow may be uniform or non - uniform, laminar or turbulent, rotational, non-rotational, steady or unsteady, one, two or three dimension.

Uniform flow is when the magnitude and direction of the velocity do not alter at any point in the fluid.
Non – uniform flow is when the velocity, pressure and depth changes in flow.

Laminar flow is when the fluid moves along in straight streamlined layers without turbulence, Fig 1 - 5
Turbulent flow is when the motion of the fluid varies rapidly in magnitude and direction at any point during the flow.

Rotational flow is when parts of the fluid rotate as the fluid flows in a circular path, and the rotation is not zero.
Non-rotational flow is when parts of the fluid stay the same as the fluid flows in a circular path, and the rotation is zero.

Steady flow is when the velocity is constant with respect with time.
Unsteady flow is complicated by changes that occur at any point with respect to time.

One dimension flow is when the direction of the velocity, temperature, pressure, density and viscosity is the same at all points.
Two-dimension flow is when the fluid movement is the same in all-parallel planes, and have gradients in two directions.
Three-dimension flow is when the flow in the fluid has gradients in three directions.

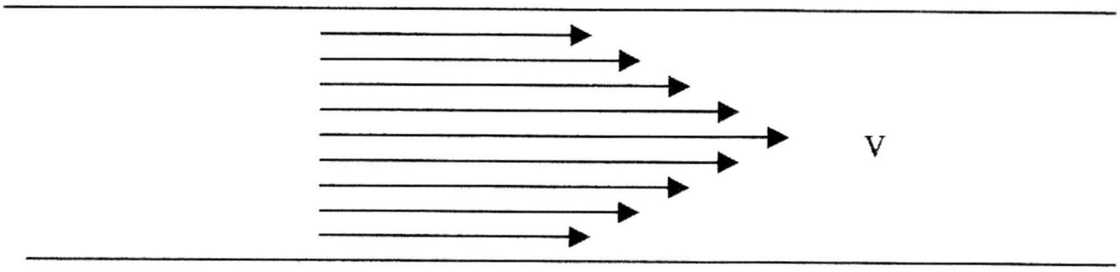

Laminar flow in a pipe

Fig. 1 – 5

Velocity of the flow is zero at the wall and increases to greatest at the centre. Fig. 1- 5

An ideal fluid is frictionless, incompressible, and free from shear stress.

Newtonian fluids are almost always liquid and gases where the shear stress is directly proportional to the transverse velocity gradient.

Non – Newtonian fluids are usually of three types –

(1) Whose properties are independent of time - or shear.
(2) Whose properties are dependant of time or shear.
(3) Exhibit characteristics of solid.

Bernoulli's equations of motion are derived from Newton's second law where the velocity of a fluid particle is assumed to be a function of time and space.
Bernoulli's equations also useful for calculating pressure change of a fluid flow from laminar flow to turbulent flow.

River System

A river channel is a path through which a fluid may flow. A closed pressurised flowing system is one that is not exposed to the atmosphere, is known as a CLOSED system – a flowing system whose surface is opened to the atmosphere, is known as an OPEN system. When a fluid flows, the process is continuous, and the mass of fluid passing a given point must remain constant – river flow depends on viscous and gravitational effects. The river is football personified.

Rivers are striking examples of a body in motion: in some cases their changes and motion have an effect on the environment, and to a certain extent a percentage of the population. Rivers are, alive, beautiful, meandering, mysterious, fast flowing and full of energy. Surface rivers are open channel dynamic system, which works from an input – output basis relying on natural springs, and rainfall to keep the system flowing. Rivers make adjustments for normal flow, and when there is an increase in input: the river responds by creating new channels – the path of least resistance to carry the water. The energy possessed by a flowing fluid consists of internal energy, and energies due to pressure, velocity, and position. When the depth varies in a river, the flow is either accelerated or retarded.
The geometry of the river system increases or decreases the resistance to flow. Specific energy of the flow is the sum of the potential and kinetic energies at a given section at the bottom of the river.

The River – Uses The Path Of Least Resistance.

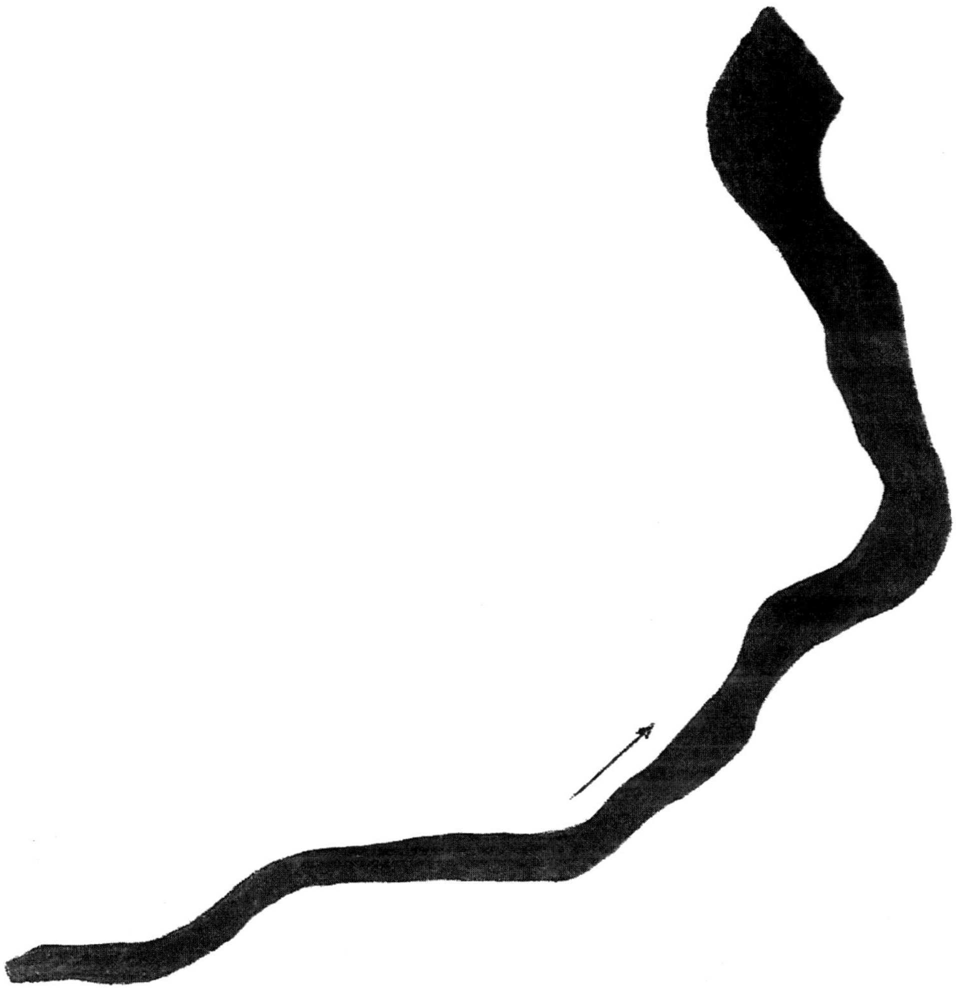

The River – an open channel flow system

Fig. 2 – 5

Imagine the players to be fluid particles in a flow. With this energised flow of the river in mind, the players will now have a mental picture of the path of least resistance which the river creates, and flows: the players can then transform this mental picture flow unto the training ground, and on match days to produce the Perfect Practice display which is exciting free flowing football – particularly, when implementing the fluent, side-foot, slide rule on the turf pass to your UNMARKED team-mate: weaving, and threading, the ball through the least congested areas – space or the path of least resistance.
The flowing river system becomes an imaginary and statutory part of the players thinking, as they look for the path of least resistance, when going forward during 90 minutes plus extra time of play.

The opponents on the other hand will try to stop this flow, by blocking the open channels – but there are open channels to create, and find: players must use them efficiently during the game: like the river.

Ball Dynamics

Ball dynamics is about, how a football – soccer ball behaves under various conditions on its own, and in relation to the player – and how the natural laws and forces of nature add a certain amount of significance for complete BALL CONTROL - and with respect for space and time AWARENESS of the game.

Ball dynamics are useful where the four dependent variables are concerned, that is, Ball Control, Passing, Possession, and the Defining Moment of the Final Ball. With some basic knowledge of ball dynamics the player will be able to work out in a split second how to control the ball with confidence to make that optimum, cross, pass or strike at goal. For example, if a ball is rising or falling, depending on the velocity, and direction of the rise, and fall – he / she needs to make the necessary adjustments to be in control of themselves, and also to be in control of the ball, before he / she strikes it correctly, and confidently.

Ball dynamics gives the player that extra amount of understanding, confidence, and edge to make the right decision, at the right time. If a player makes a mistake, and strikes the ball incorrectly or at the wrong moment – he / she will know instantly, why the ball did not go to the target it was intended for.

Gravitation

Gravitation is a universal law discovered by Newton, and states that all bodies in the universe attract each other. Where people are concerned, the attraction between each other is not noticeable, because of the great mass of the earth in comparison to the small masses created by people. Ocean and sea tides are caused by the gravitational pulls of the sun and moon, acting alternately, together, and in opposition.

Gravitational Variations – and Acceleration due to Gravity

In Europe, a ball of mass 0.25 kilograms weighs 0.25x 9.81=2.45 N, The letter N denotes Newton but at the equatorial region, it may be 2.20 N. This is due to the earth's rotation, and the earth not being a complete sphere. Gravitational force is greater at the north, and south poles, than the equator. 1newton N = 0.101 kg. 9.81 is the acceleration due to gravity – calculated from 1gm. Wt.= 1 x 9.81= 9.81 dynes or 9.81 metres per second per second or 32 ft per sec per sec., and is denoted by the letter g – for a freely falling body, the weight or force produces a downward uniform acceleration.

Force

A force is defined as a physical effort, which can change the rest or motion of an object. A force must be applied to a body, to change its state of rest, to a state of motion – for example, a footballer taking a penalty, is from a ball at rest to a ball in motion. To increase a footballer's velocity – for example, if a player is running at 1 metre / second and wants to get up to 2 metres / second, he / she will have to run faster.

To change the direction of motion of a player – for example, if a player is running in one direction and then suddenly changes, a force has to be applied to slow the player down, before he/she changes direction.

The different types of forces are – accelerating, retarding, attractive, repulsion, and resistive forces.

The force is represented by the Newton N, and is defined as – that force when applied to a mass of one kilogram gives an acceleration of one metre per second per second.

1N = 1 kg metres per second per second

The force required to produce an acceleration or retardation of a body, is the product of the mass in kilograms multiplied by the acceleration in metres per second.

F is the force in Newton
a = the acceleration in metres per second per second
m= the mass of the body

Then F = ma from Newton's second law - page 50

A footballer has a mass of 70 kilograms, and accelerates at 2 metres per second per second. What force is produced by the footballer?

Applying the formula

F = ma
F = 70 x 2
F = 140 N

Gravity and Weight

Gravity is defined as the gravitational force, between one planet, and a body on its surface, within its gravitational field. Gravity is responsible for the weight of a body – it is the force exerted by the planet on that body.

Weight

Weight is defined as the force of attraction of the earth on a given mass, and varies according to its geographical location. The weight of an object can be measured using a spring balance and noting the extension – the extension is proportional to the force acting on it.

If a ball of mass 0.30 kg falls from the top of the goal bar – it falls with an acceleration of 9.81 metres per second per second. What is the force produced?

Applying the formula

F = ma
F = 0.30 x 9.81
F = 2.95 N

Mass

Mass is defined as the quantity of matter in that body, and is the same regardless of its geographical location.

Calculate the mass of a football of weight 3.0 N.

Weight of ball = 3.0 N
mass x 9.81 = 3.0
Therefore mass = $\frac{3.0}{9.81}$
The mass of the ball = 0.30 kg

The S.I. Unit of mass is the kilogram.

The mass of the earth is approximately 5.976×10^{24} kg

Equilibrium – Centre of Gravity and Toppling

Equilibrium – when a body is at rest, all the forces that act upon it, balance each other and there are three states of equilibrium.

(1) Stable
(2) Unstable
(3) Neutral

(1) Stable equilibrium – if a body is at rest, and is slightly displaced, it tends to return to its original position, example - a block resting on one of its sides.
(2) Unstable equilibrium – when an object is displaced, it tends to move away from its original position, example – a spinning top at the end of its spin – or a footballer leaning backwards far too much. Fig. 3 – 5 (c).
(3) Neutral equilibrium – when an object is moved, and is centre of gravity is not changed, example – a ball resting on its sides.

Centre of Gravity and Toppling

Centre of gravity and toppling are very useful to the footballer when striking a ball, as you will discover later, and in your Perfect Practice. If you support a ruler on your forefinger, and adjust it, so that it is balanced, then the centre of gravity of the ruler is the point where the forefinger supports the ruler, without it falling to either side. It is the fixed point through which the resultant force of gravity always passes, not taking into account the position of the body.

If a player stands upright, he / she will not topple over, because his / her centre of gravity is not altered – if the player leans forward, backwards, or sideways, to an extent which alters his / her centre of gravity greatly, the player will topple over.
An imaginary vertical line drawn through the centre of gravity of a body is called a line of direction of the body – so long as the line of direction falls within the base of the body: the body will stand – when the line of direction falls outside the base of the body – the body will topple or fall over.

Fig. 3 – 5 shows three players –

(a) The player is standing upright – as the vertical line drawn through O falls within the base AB, the player will not topple over.
(b) The player is leaning slightly backwards, but the vertical line drawn through O is still within the base AB, and the player will not topple over.
(c) The player is leaning even further backwards - the vertical line drawn through O falls outside the base AB, and the player will topple or fall over.

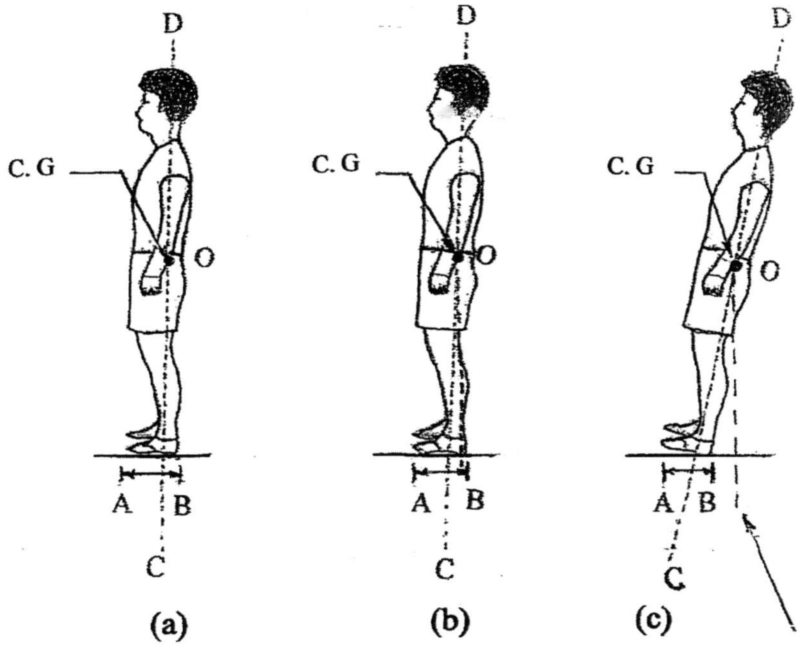

Fig. 3 – 5

In Fig. 4 – 5, if a player takes a penalty or strikes the final ball towards goal by leaning further back, as the "lean back" is indicated in Fig. 3 – 5 (c) where the centre of gravity vertical line is outside the base AB – the ball will rise over the bar and if, the ball is already rising when struck, it will go even higher over the bar; this can happen quite close up to the goalmouth, even as close as 3 metres – so players must get the DEFINING MOMENT OF THE FINAL BALL RIGHT to avoid lifting the ball over the bar.

Do not lean backwards when striking the ball near the goal mouth – only when the player is a long way off goal, and needs to lift the ball, to get underneath it the player should lean backwards, like making an over the top cross or pass.

The correct way to strike an on the turf ball is shown in Fig. 5 – 5. For an on the turf acute angle strike where the player's head is down, the centre of gravity is within the player's base, and the side of the foot is used to kick the ball - are included in the production of the DEFINING MOMENT OF THE FINAL BALL for this type of strike, and other strikes in Chapter 6.
The vertical or slightly forward centre of gravity tilt in line with its base helps the player to get on top of the ball to keep it down.
The backward centre of gravity tilt helps the player to get beneath the ball to give the ball lift – the degree of backward lean of the centre of gravity line to outside its base will give the desired lift of the ball required by the player. When running with or without the ball, if the player is at maximum velocity and the player's lean angle becomes too forward at any point in time during the run the player will topple and fall-over: so a compromise between velocity and balance must be reached to avoid falling over.

So, when a player misses a sitter in front of goal from a relatively close distance – he / she will immediately know why the ball went over the bar or wide of the post – then take corrective measures to prevent it from happening again as described.

Unrestricted Centre of Gravity of the Striker

Fig. 4 – 5 the striker's centre of gravity is outside his / her base at impact with the ball, so the ball is given more lift, by getting under the ball, and it goes over the bar.

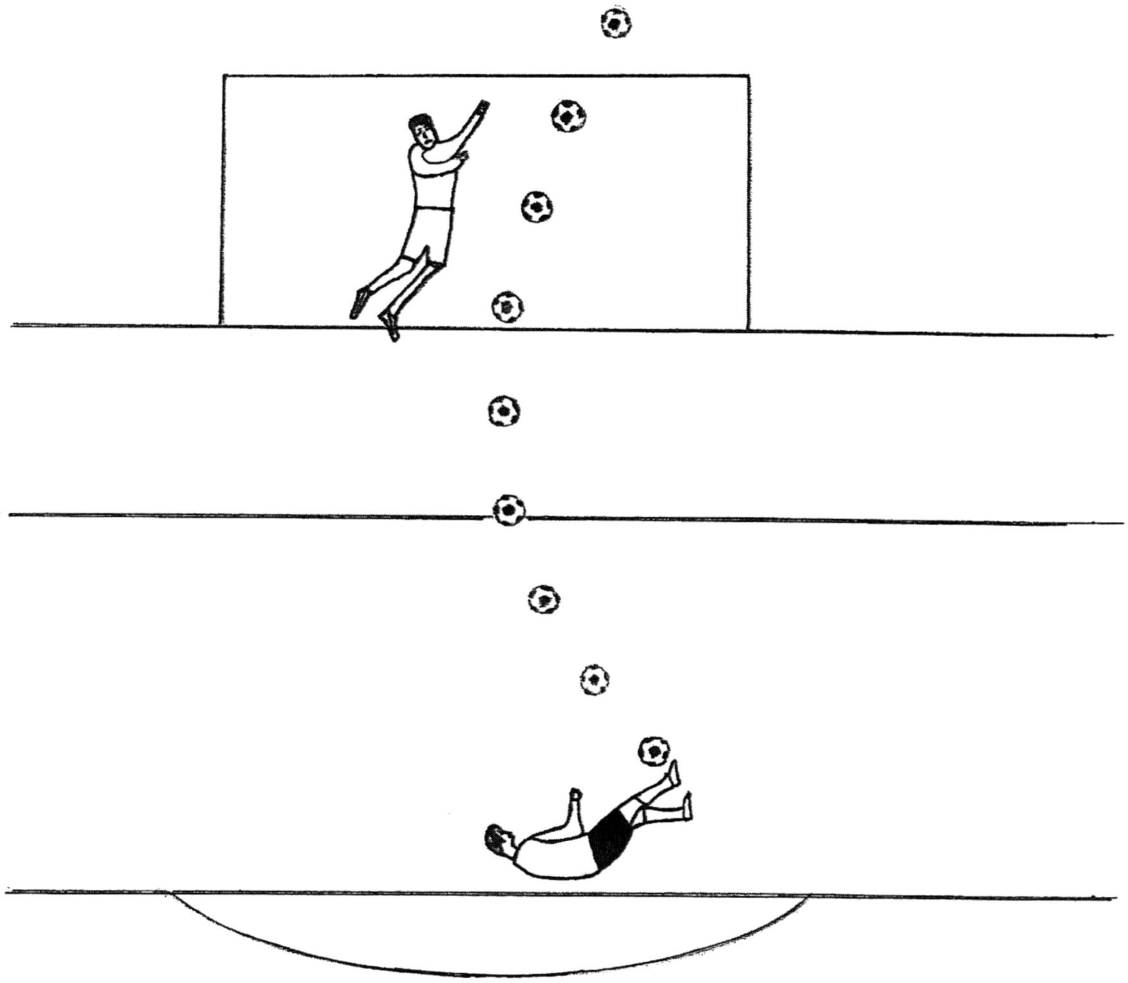

Restricted Centre of Gravity of the Striker

Fig. 5 – 5 the striker's centre of gravity is within his / her base which gives the correct body posture for implementing the DEFINING MOMENT OF THE FINAL BALL - in the horizontal plane – on the turf.

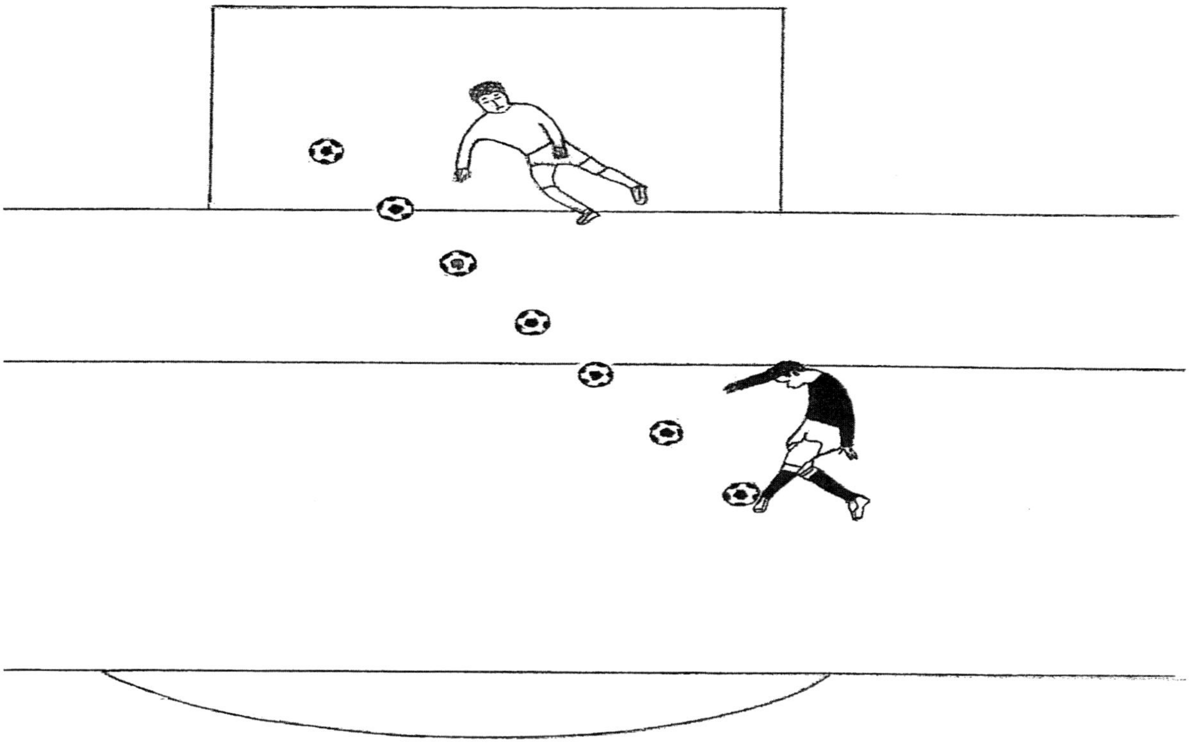

To calculate the approximate centre of gravity of the average footballer / soccer player - consider Fig. 6 – 5 where the larger rectangle A_1 represents the player's body and the smaller rectangle, A_2 represents the player's head with average dimensions. We know the centre of gravity of each rectangle, because they are symmetrical, and use weight is proportional to area to calculate the distance x from C – also the centre of gravity will lie along the line.

C O at a distance x from C

Taking moments about C

Area of $A_1 = 60 \text{ X } 160 = 9600 \text{ cm}^2$

Area of $A_2 = 15 \text{ X } 20 = 300\text{cm}^2$

Use the formula –

$A_1 \times 80 + A_2 \times 170 = (A_1 + A_2)\, x$
$(9600 \times 80) + (300 \times 170) = (9600 + 300)\, x$
$768000 + 51000 = (9600 + 300)\, x$
$819000 = (9900)\, x$
$x = \frac{819000}{9900}$
$x = 82.72 \text{ cm from A}$

But other body parts such as the arms, etc., must be compensated for - and an additional 20% / 30% of 82.72 cm – that is, 20% /30% extra body weight.

$\frac{30}{100} \times 82.72 = 24.81$

24.81 + 82.72 = 107.53 cm or near because of varying build and weights of players.

The centre of gravity of the average footballer / soccer player is approximately 107.53 cm from the sole of the feet to around the navel, and near the spine in line with the heel of the feet.

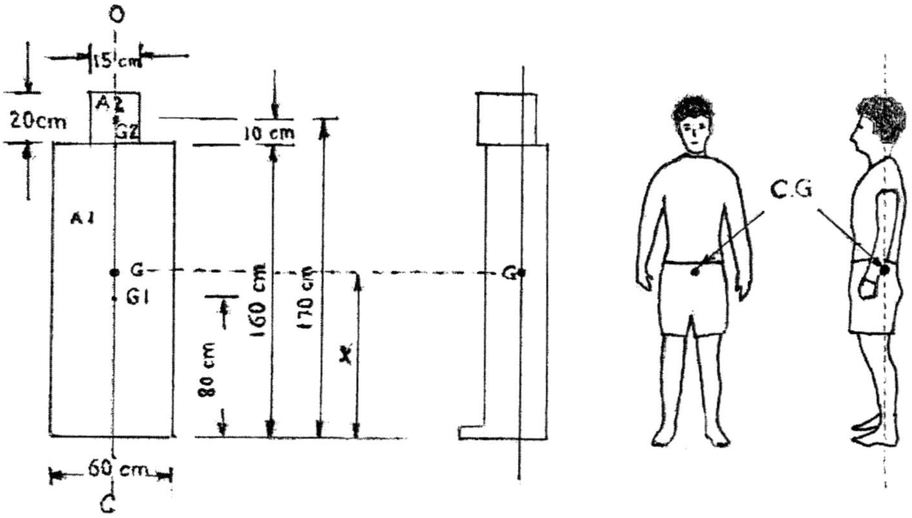

Fig 6 – 5

Motion

Motion is defined as change of position of a body, for example, if a ball is rolling down a hill, it is in motion in relation to the hill.

There are three types of motion –

(1) Rectilinear motion – motion in a straight-line.
(2) Curvature, curvilinear, space curve, or curve path motion.
(3) Circular motion, see angular velocity.

(1) Fig. 7 – 5 shows rectilinear motion or motion in a straight line of a ball moving from one position to the next. This continuous motion and the direction remaining unchanged produce a rectilinear or straight-line motion.
(2) Fig. 8 – 5 shows the curvature of a curve at a point P on it, is the rate at which the direction changes for a given length.

Curvature, curvilinear, space curve or curve path motion of a ball is a small straight line broken between one line and the next; but the direction of the line changes at each broken point following the other - moment of inertia, and drag forces oppose Newton's first law of motion which causes the line to break, and change direction. Continuous change in the direction of these broken lines produces a curve path as in the case of a football / soccer ball, Fig. 8 -5.

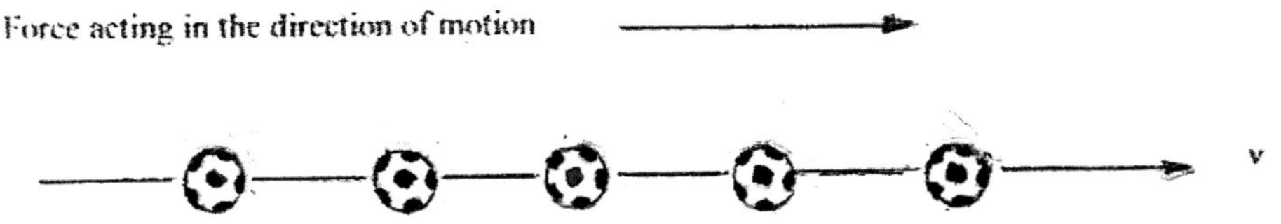

Fig. 7 – 5 rectilinear or straight-line motion

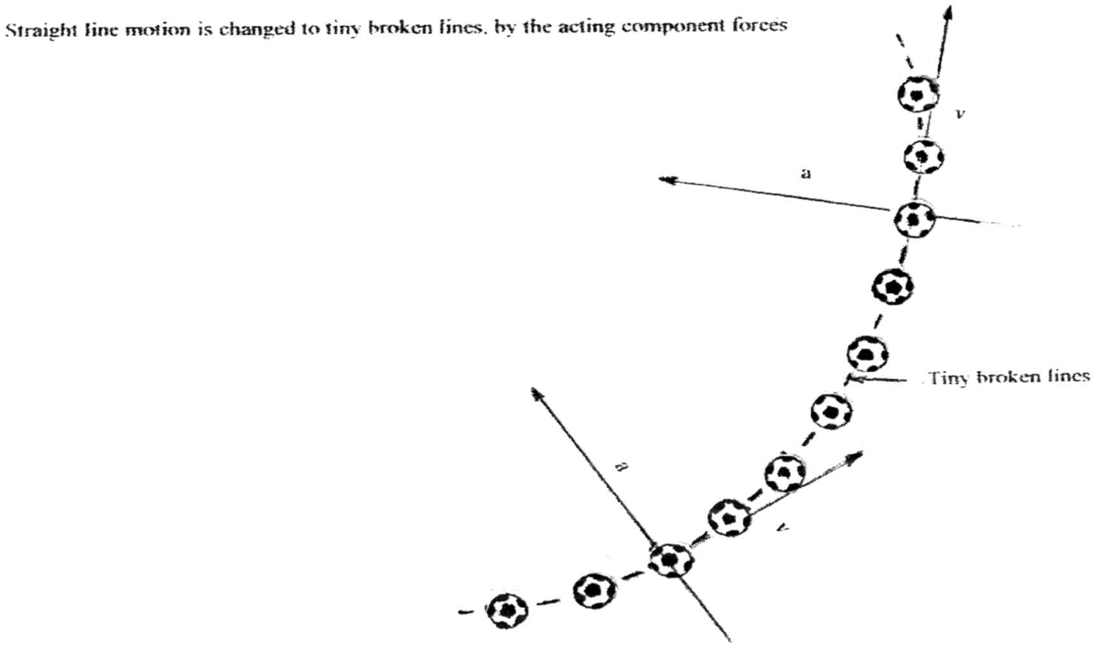

Curvilinear motion
Fig. 8 – 5

Derived Units - Dimensions

The units used for - velocity - and acceleration are obtained from the derived units of dimension. For speed and velocity – the fundamental units of length and time represented by L and T of dimensions 1 and - 1 respectively which gives L T: so the unit for velocity used in this manual is $m\,s^{-1}$.
For acceleration – the units of L and T have dimensions 1 and -2 respectively, which gives L T: so the unit for acceleration used in this manual is $m\,s^{-2}$.

Speed – Velocity – Acceleration

Speed

Speed is defined as the ratio of distance to time – speed has magnitude, and is a scalar quantity with units of $m\ s^{-1}$.

$$\text{speed} = \frac{\text{distance}}{\text{time}}$$

$$\text{distance} = \text{speed x time}$$

$$\text{time} = \frac{\text{distance}}{\text{speed}}$$

If a footballer covers a distance of 70 metres in 12 seconds, what is the speed of the footballer?

$$\text{speed} = \frac{70}{12}$$

$$\text{speed} = 5.83\ m\ s^{-1}$$

Velocity

Velocity is defined as the rate of motion in a given direction, measured as distance v time. Velocity can be expressed in centimetres per second – metres per second – kilometres per hour – feet per second – and miles per hour.
Velocity has magnitude, as well as direction: a vector quantity.

Uniform Velocity

Uniform velocity of a body is when equal distances are covered in equal times: that is, its motion is constant.

Uniformly Varying Velocity

Uniformly varying velocity of a body is when the velocity varies – that is, retarded or accelerated.

Average Velocity of a body is calculated during a specified time, for example, if a player is moving at a velocity of $2\ m\ s^{-1}$ and 3 seconds later, he / she is moving at $5\ m\ s^{-1}$ the distance covered in the 3 seconds period, will be the same, as if the player were moving with a uniform velocity of: $\frac{2+5}{2} = 3.5\ m\ s^{-1}$

Equations of Velocity – Distance – Time

Letters are allocated to the relationship of velocity, distance, and time as follows:

v = velocity
s = distance
t = time

$$v = \frac{s}{t}$$

$$s = v\,t$$

$$t = \frac{s}{v}$$

Conversion of Units

Sometimes it may be necessary to convert one unit into another, for example, to convert 5 kilometres per hour into metres per second – multiply 5 by 1000 metres and divide by 3600 seconds: 1 kilometre = 1000 metres and 1 hour = 3600 seconds.

$$\frac{5 \times 1000}{3600}$$
$$= 1.38 \text{ m s}^{-1} \text{ or}$$

Convert 5 miles per hour into feet per second – multiply 5 by 5280 feet, and divide by 3600 seconds equals:

$$\frac{5 \times 5280}{3600}$$
$$= 7.3 \text{ ft s}^{-1}.$$

Values must be expressed in their proper units, depending on how the values are given, and what is asked for, if the velocity is in km / h, the distance must be in kilometres and the time in hours.

Velocity – Worked Examples

Some worked examples to give the players a clearer picture of how a few problems are approached.

A midfield player runs down the middle of the pitch with a velocity of 7 m s^{-1}. What distance he / she cover in 5 seconds.

Applying $s = v\,t$
$s = 7 \times 5$
$s = 35\text{m}$

If a winger runs down the right flank with the ball and covers a distance of 40 metres in 5 seconds. What is the velocity of the winger?

Applying $v = \frac{s}{t}$

$v = \frac{40}{5}$

$v = 8\ m\ s^{-1}$

If a centre forward has a uniform velocity of $5\ m\ s^{-1}$. How long will it take the centre forward to cover a distance of 50 metres?

Applying $t = \frac{s}{v}$

$t = \frac{50}{5}$

$t = 10\ s$

Acceleration and Retardation – straight- line or linear

Acceleration is defined as the rate of change of velocity. When a force is applied to a free moving body, the velocity of the body changes, and if the force applied is variable, and continues to act the velocity will be variable. The magnitude of the velocity will depend on the amount of force that is applied for a given time - the quantity, and direction of the force will tell whether the velocity, is increasing, or decreasing with respect to time.

For example, suppose a centre half starts from rest, and gets at a uniform rate to a velocity of 7 meters per second in a time of 7 seconds, the centre half will have an acceleration of 7 meters per second per second in a time of 7 seconds – that is, the change of velocity is 1 meter per second for each second.

Uniform or Constant Acceleration – is produced by a uniform or a constant force.

Retardation

Retardation is the opposite of acceleration, where a force is applied to a body to slow it down- negative sign.

If a player is running at velocity of $7\ m\ s^{-1}$, then slows down to $4\ m\ s^{-1}$, the player has undergone retardation.

Speed – Velocity – Acceleration and Retardation – requires good control

Are useful to the player where running with the ball, and not over-hitting or under-hitting, so as to keep possession – out running the opponents, getting to the ball first to win the ball, to keep possession – change of pace to surprise, confuse the opponents, and get away rapidly from opponents.

A player cannot exceed his / her maximum acceleration or velocity, when running with the ball or without the ball at that point in time. The player cannot give what he / she do not have. There are limits as to how fast players could run, but there will be players who are faster than others in either acceleration, velocity, or both and also some players could slow down more quickly than others – retardation: also control of the player's centre of gravity has to be taken into account in running.

Equations of Motion

To develop the three equations of motion, to solve different types of problems involving players, and ball: consider that uniform acceleration is the change of velocity in a unit of time – this is found by dividing the total change of velocity by the time the change takes place.

Using letter notations –

a = acceleration
u = velocity at the beginning of interval
v = velocity at end of interval
t = time interval

If the velocity of a striker moving in a straight line with a uniform acceleration a, increases from a value u, to a value v, in a time t, thus, from definition of acceleration –

$$a = \frac{v - u}{t}$$

change the formula to give v

$$v = u + at \text{ ....equation (1)}$$

If a player is moving with uniform acceleration, his / her average velocity is equal to half the sum of the initial velocity u, and the final v. The next two equations of motion require the evaluation of average velocity, distance, and time.

Therefore the average velocity –

$$= \frac{u + v}{2}$$

but v = u + at from equation (1)

$$\text{average velocity} = \frac{u + u + at}{2}$$

$$\text{average velocity} = u + \frac{1}{2} at$$

The distance s travelled = average velocity x time

$$s = (u + \frac{1}{2} at) t$$

$$s = u t + \frac{1}{2} at^2 \text{ ....equation (2)}$$

To find t from equation (1) and changing the subject of the formula

$$t = \frac{v - u}{a}$$

Substitution of t in equation (2) gives

$$s = u \frac{(v - u)}{a} + \frac{1}{2} a \frac{(v - u)}{a}^2$$

$$s = \frac{v - u}{a}\left[u + \frac{1}{2}a\frac{(v - u)}{a}\right]$$

$$s = \frac{v - u}{a}\left[\frac{2u + v - u}{2}\right]$$

$$2as = (v - u)(v + a) = v^2 - u^2$$

$$v^2 - u^2 = 2\,as \text{......................equation (3)}$$

Worked Examples

(1) A football is kicked vertically upwards with an initial velocity of 15 m s^{-1}. Calculate the time taken for the ball to reach the top of its motion.

This can be found from equation (1)

$$v = u + at$$

The velocity at the top of its motion is zero and
since $u = 15$, and $a = - 9.81$

we get $0 = 15 – 9.81\ t$

$$t = \frac{15}{9.81}$$

$$t = 1.53\ s$$

(2) The right winger runs down the flank, with a velocity of 5 m s^{-1}. The velocity has uniform acceleration and at the end of 5 seconds reaches 8 m s^{-1}. What is the acceleration of the winger?

Use equation (1)

$v = u + at$

$u = 5\ m\ s^{-1}$

$v = 8\ m\ s^{-1}$

$t = 5\ s$

$a = ?$

therefore

$8 = 5 + a\ 5$

$3 = a\ 5$

$$a = \frac{3}{5}\ m\ s^{-2}$$

The right winger's acceleration $= \frac{3}{5}\ m\ s^{-2}$

(2) If a striker starts from rest – from the half way line, towards the opponent goal, and reaches a velocity of 8 kilometres per hour in 4 seconds. (a) What is the striker's acceleration? (b) What distance is covered in the first 7 seconds? - assuming his / her acceleration stays uniform during that time.

(a)

Let $u = 0$
$v = 8$ km / hr
$t = 7$ s
$a = ?$

Convert kilometres per hour to metres per second.
Therefore 8 kilometres per hour is equal to,

$$\frac{8000}{3600} = 2.2 \text{ m s}^{-1}$$

Using $v = u + at$

$$2.2 = 0 + 4a$$

$$a = \frac{2.2}{4}$$

$$a = 0.55 \text{ m s}^{-2}.$$

The striker's acceleration is
$= 0.55 \text{ m s}^{-2}$.

(b)

Let
$a = 0.55 \text{ m s}^{-2}$
$t = 7$ s
$u = 0$
$s = ?$

Using $s = ut + \frac{1}{2}at^2$

$$s = 0 + \frac{1}{2} \times 0.55 \times 49$$

$$s = 13.5\text{m}.$$

The distance covered in the first 7 seconds is
$= 13.5$ m.

(3) How long will it take a midfield player, to cover 70 metres if he / she accelerates uniformly from rest with the ball, and keeping pace with it, at the rate of 2 m s^{-2}

Let $s = 70$ m
$u = 0$
$a = 2 \text{ m s}^{-2}$
$t = ?$

Using $s = ut + \frac{1}{2}at^2$

$$70 = 0 + \frac{1}{2} \times 2t^2$$

$2t^2 = 140$

$t^2 = \frac{140}{2}$

then $t = \sqrt{\frac{140}{2}}$ therefore t = 8.4 s

The time taken by the striker to cover 70 metres is
= 8.4 s.

(4) A right winger accelerates down the flank uniformly from rest with the ball at is feet - at the rate of 0.3 m s^{-2}. What is the velocity of the winger after covering a distance of 50 metres?

Let $u = 0$
$a = 0.3 m s^{-2}$
$s = 50 m$
$v = ?$

Using $v^2 - u^2 = 2 a s$
$v^2 - 0 = 0.3 x 2 x 50$
$v^2 = 30$
$v = \sqrt{30}$
$v = 5.47 m s^{-1}$

(5) A football is kicked vertically upwards to a height of 25 metres.
How long will it take the ball to strike the ground?

Let $u = 0$
$a = g = 9.81 m s^{-2}$
$s = 25 m$
$t = ?$

Using $s = u t + \frac{1}{2} a t^2$

$25 = 0 + \frac{1}{2} x 9.81 t^2$

$t^2 = \frac{2 x 50}{9.81}$

$t = \sqrt{\frac{100}{9.81}}$

$= 3.19 s$

The Dynamics of Projectiles

A football kicked upwards, at an angle to the horizontal – or headed a certain distance above the horizontal, at an angle or horizontally is called a projectile.

A projectile has a downward acceleration due to gravity g. The horizontal velocity stays constant because there is no natural force acting in this direction. In solving problems of this nature, the two components are calculated separately.

The horizontal motion is considered first, and then the vertical motion second.

The dynamics of projectiles are useful to the footballer in enabling him or her to understand the angles, time, and range, for directional control of the ball with head or feet, on the turf or off the turf – for example, providing a slide rule over the top cross or pass to an UNMARKED team-mate, provide a knock down header to an UNMARKED team-mate: a knock down header for a scramble in the opponent 18 yd / penalty area to chip the opponent keeper or to score directly into the opponent net.
In defence to clear the ball out of dangerous areas quickly, decisively, and safely using the head or feet to do so.

In Chapter 6 on ball control - passing - possession and the final ball, trigonometry was applied to calculate the various distances, and angles of the ball on or above the turf. In this Chapter – in addition to angles and distances – velocity, acceleration, and time, are involved in the calculations in the various angled balls on or above the turf: to show a wider relationship between angles, distances, velocity, acceleration, and time with respect to the footballers using time, and space awareness effectively, and to enhance the accuracy of directional control of the ball.

Worked Examples

In the following worked examples – when a football is kicked at an angle of elevation θ to the horizontal or headed horizontally at eye level – headed downwards, below eye level: the angle of depression – headed upwards above eye level - acute angle – both the horizontal and vertical motions must be calculated individually. Write down the details of what is known – what is unknown, and what is required using the statutory notations, and applying the appropriate formulae: in some cases the formulae will have to be re-arranged to find the unknown or what is required.
The horizontal velocity u cos θ is constant and the vertical velocity u sin θ is affected by gravity g.

Fig. 9 – 5 shows the various projectile angles most commonly used by the footballer,

Various Projectile Angles With Respect to the Turf – The Horizontal Plane and Above the Turf – The Vertical Plane

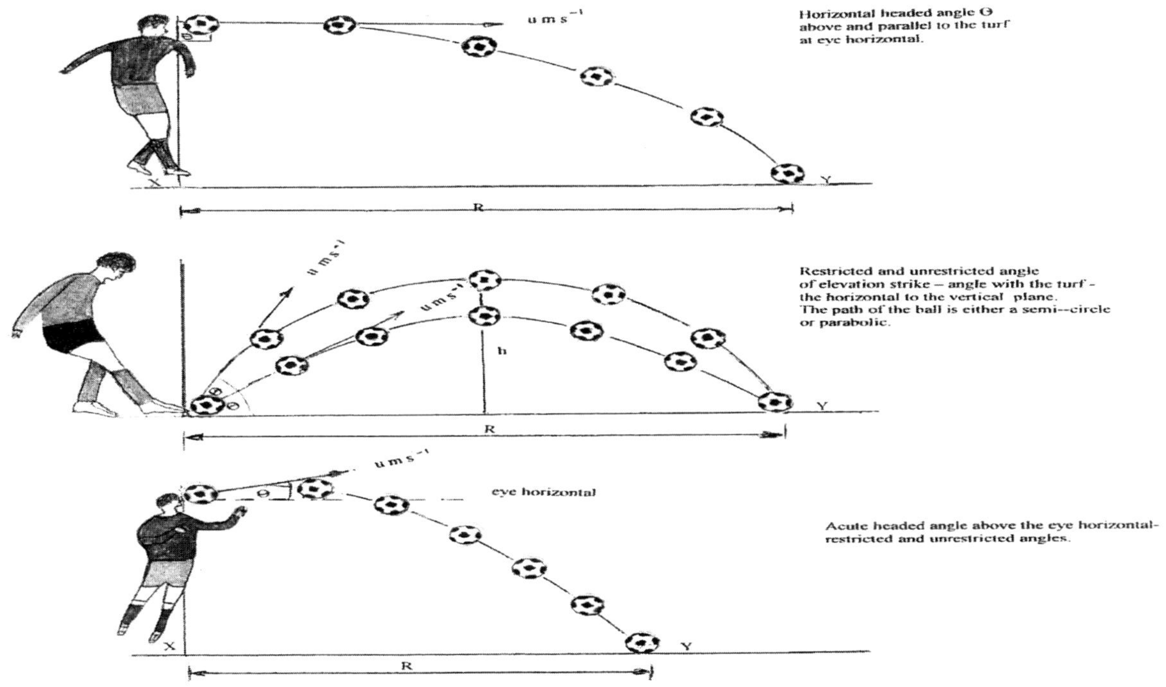

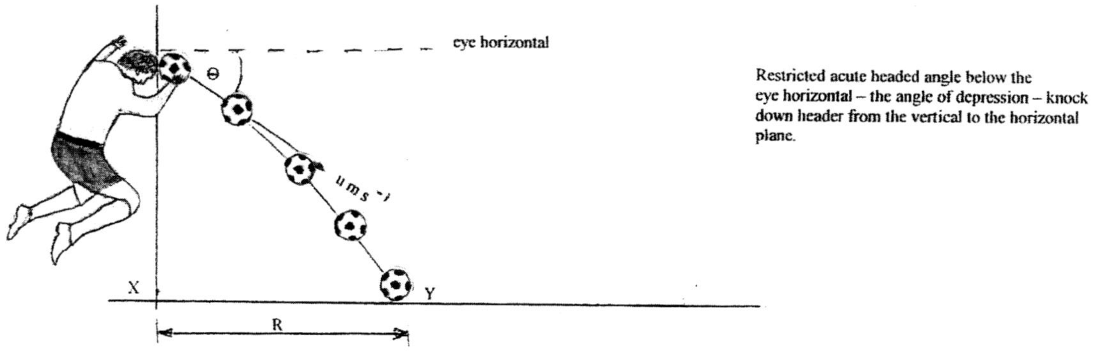

Fig. 9 –5

Example 1

A centre back kicks a football with an initial velocity of 30 m s^{-1} at an angle of elevation of 40° to the horizontal.
Calculate (a) the highest point attained by the ball.
(b) the time taken for the ball to reach the highest point.

Details of horizontal motion.

$u = 30 \cos 40^o$ m s^{-1}
$s = d$
$t = t$
$a = 0$

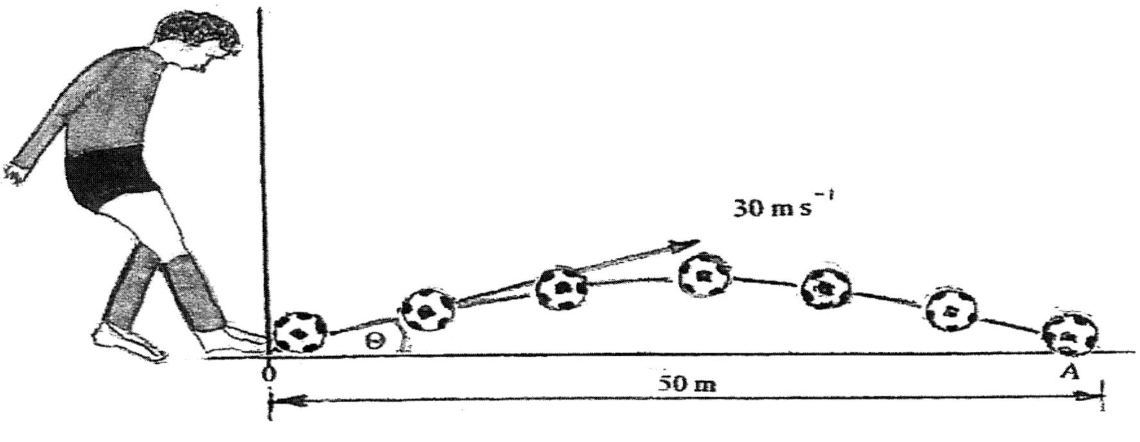

Fig 10 – 5

Details of vertical motion.

$u = 30 \sin 40^o$ m s^{-1}

$s = h$
$v = 0$
$a = -9.81 \text{ m s}^{-2}$
$t = t$

For vertical motion to find the highest point use $v^2 = u^2 + 2as$ substitute h for s in the equation.

$0 = (30 \sin 40^{o}) + 2(-9.81)\,h$
$= (30 \times 0.642) + 19.62\,h$
$h = \dfrac{(30 \times 0.642)}{19.62}$
$= 18.9 \text{ m}$

For vertical motion to find the time use

$v = u + a\,t$
$0 = 30 \sin 40^{o} + (-9.81)\,t$
$t = \dfrac{30 \sin 40^{o}}{9.81}$
$t = \dfrac{19.26}{9.81}$
$t = 1.9 \text{ s}$

The highest point reached by the ball is 18.9 m and the time is 1.9 s

Example 2

A centre back makes an over the top pass at a velocity of 30 m s^{-1} to an UNMARKED team-mate in splendid isolation 50 metres away.
Calculate the angle of elevation θ to the horizontal of the football.

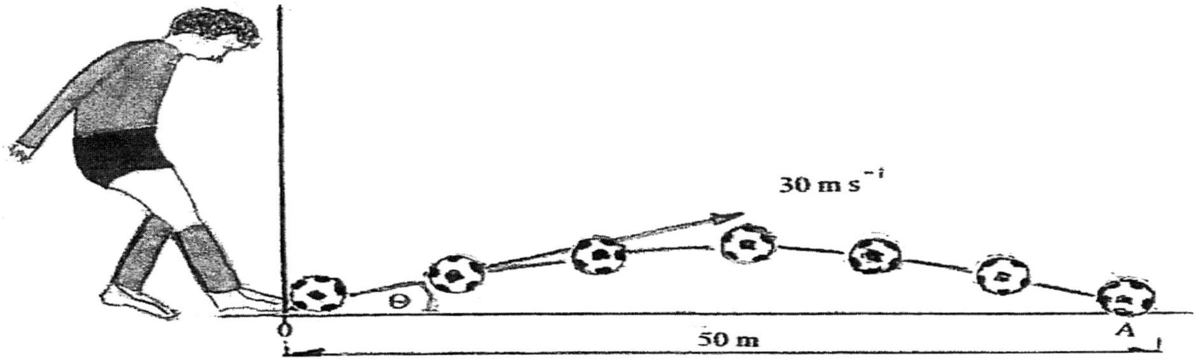

Fig. 11 – 5

Details of horizontal motion.

$u = 30 \cos \theta \text{ m s}^{-1}$
$s = 50 \text{ m}$
$t = t$
$a = 0$

Details of vertical motion

$u = 30 \sin \theta \text{ m s}^{-1}$
$s = 0$

$t = t$
$a = 9.81\ m\ s^{-2}$

To find the time for vertical motion use –

$$s = ut + \frac{1}{2}at^2$$

$$0 = (30 \sin\theta)t - \frac{1}{2}(9.81)t^2$$

At O t = zero

$$t = 2\left(\frac{30 \sin\theta}{9.81}\right) \text{ at A}$$

To find the angle use –
Distance = velocity x time for horizontal motion, and the standard
Trig,. identity $\sin 2\theta = 2\sin\theta\cos\theta$

distance = velocity x time.

$$50 = 30 \cos\theta \times 60 \frac{\sin\theta}{9.81}$$

Trig,. identity

$$\sin 2\theta = \frac{50 \times 9.81}{30 \times 30}$$
$$= 0.54$$
$$2\theta = 33^o$$
$$\theta = 16.5^o$$

Example 3

A right winger kicks a football at an angle of elevation of 20° to the horizontal, and with an initial velocity of $25\ m\ s^{-1}$. His / her team-mate is moving into the opponent 18 yd / penalty area, to receive the over the top pass. Calculate (a) How long will it take the ball to reach his / her team-mate? (b) How far away his / her team-mate has to be in order to receive the ball?
(a)

The motion of the football in the range OA Fig 12 - 5

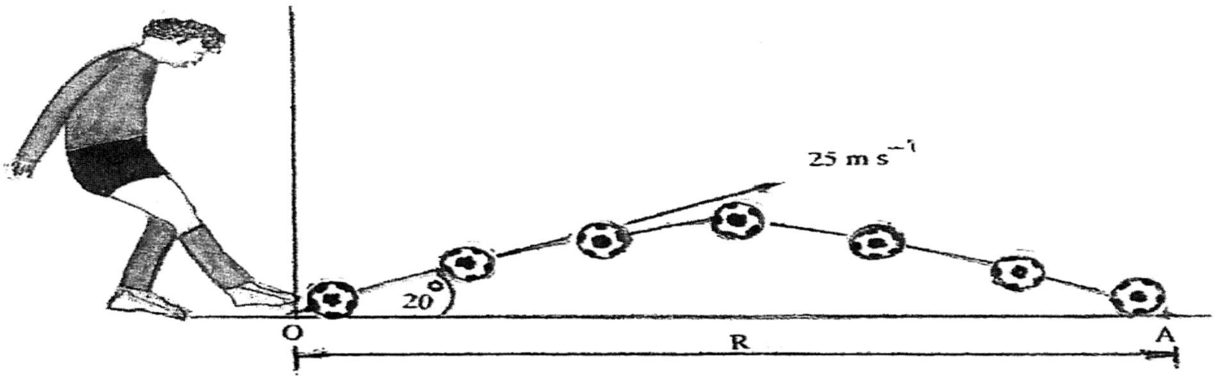

Details of horizontal motion

$u = 25 \cos \theta \text{ m s}^{-1}$
$s = R$
$t = t$
$a = 0$

Details of vertical motion

$u = 25 \sin \theta \text{ m s}^{-1}$
$s = 0$
$t = t$
$a = 9.81 \text{ m s}^{-2}$

For vertical motion to find the time use –

$$s = ut + \frac{1}{2}at^2$$

$$0 = (25 \sin 20^o)\, t - \frac{1}{2}(9.81)\, t^2$$

$$t = \frac{8.55 \times 2}{9.81}$$

$$t = 1.7 \text{ s}$$

(b)

For horizontal motion to find the distance or range use –
Distance = velocity x time

$$s = 25 \times 1.7$$
$$= 42.5 \text{ m}$$

The time for the ball to reach his / her team–mate is 1.7 s
The distance his / her team–mate has to be is 42.5 m

Example 4

Horizontal and Maximum Range

Horizontal Range

This type of angle of elevation kick – useful when an opposing goalkeeper is off his / her line or out of his / her goal area, and cannot get back in time to stop the ball from going in the net.

If a football is kicked with an initial velocity u, at an angle of elevation θ to the horizontal – the component in a horizontal direction is u cos θ and the component in a vertical direction is u sin θ.
Using $v = u + at$ and

$$s = ut + \frac{1}{2}at^2$$

$$a = -g$$

The vertical velocity v of the ball in a time t is

$v = \sin\theta - gt$

The vertical distance s of the ball in a time t

$s = u \sin\theta \times t - \frac{1}{2} gt^2$

The vertical velocity of the ball at the highest point is zero.

Therefore $\theta = \sin\theta - gt^2$

t is the time for the ball to reach the highest point

$t = \frac{u \sin\theta}{g}$

When the ball hits the ground at A - the vertical distance travelled is zero.

Using $o = u \sin\theta \times t - \frac{1}{2} gt^2$ to find the time

$t = 2 \frac{u \sin\theta}{g}$

The range of the ball is the horizontal distance OA which is the horizontal velocity x time.

$= u \cos\theta \times 2 \frac{u \sin\theta}{g}$

$= \frac{u^2 \sin\theta}{g}$

Maximum Range

To produce a maximum range – the optimum angle of kick – the angle of elevation should be 45° to the horizontal.

The maximum value of $\sin\theta = 1$

$2\theta = 90^o$

$\theta = 45^o$ for a given value of u.

The smaller the angle – the flight time becomes quicker due to a larger horizontal component of the velocity u – also the shortest distance between two points is a straight line.

Example 1

A goalkeeper kicks a football over the top at an angle of elevation of 60° to the horizontal with an initial velocity of 30 m s^{-1}.

Calculate (a) The horizontal range – of the football.

(b) The maximum range – of the football.

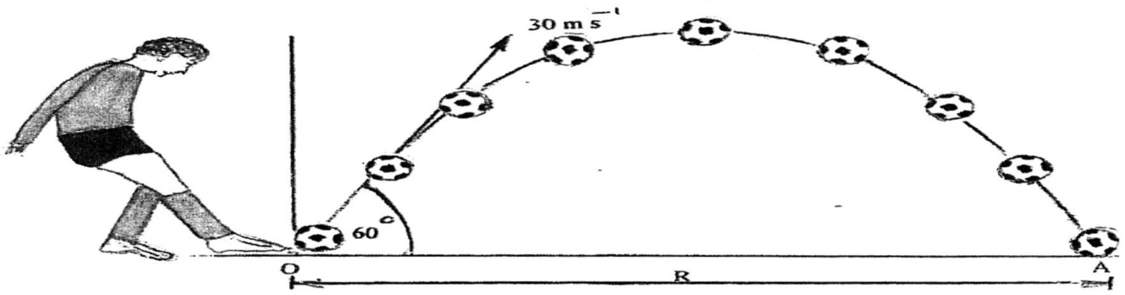

Fig. 13 - 5

(a) The horizontal range

$u = 30\ \text{m s}^{-1}$

$\theta = 60^{o}$

Using $R = \dfrac{30^{2} \sin \theta}{9.81}$

$= 79.45$ m

(b) The maximum range

$R\ max. = \dfrac{u^{2}}{g}$ when $\theta = 45^{o}$

$R\ max = \dfrac{30^{2}}{9.81}$

$= 91.7$ m

Horizontal Header – Above and Parallel to the Turf Surface

Example 1

A football is headed in a horizontal direction, at a velocity of $25\ \text{m s}^{-1}$ by a leaping centre forward from a height of approximately 2.5 m off and parallel to the turf surface.

Calculate (a) the time taken for the ball to hit the turf.

(b) the distance a team-mate has to be in order to receive the ball in that time.

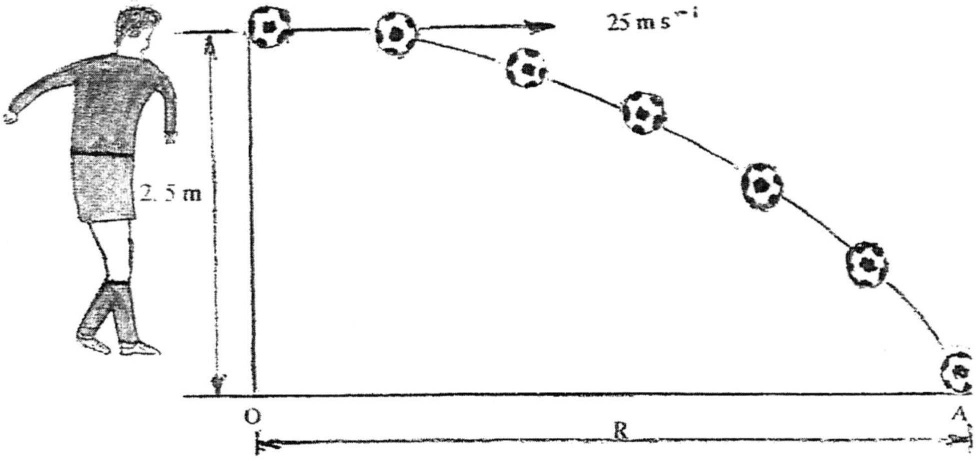

Fig. 14 –5

Details for horizontal motion

$u = 25\ \text{m s}^{-1}$

$s = x$
$t = t$
$a = 0$

Details for vertical motion

$u = 0$
$s = 2.5$ m
$t = t$
$a = 9.81 \text{ m s}^{-2}$

To find the time when the ball hits the turf for vertical motion -

Use $s = ut + \frac{1}{2}at^2$

$2.5 = 0 + \frac{1}{2}(9.81)\,t^2$

$t^2 = \frac{2\,(2.5)}{9.81}$

$t = \sqrt{0.50}$

$t = 0.71$ s

To find the distance where the ball hits the ground, and reaches the team-mate,
Use distance = velocity x time

$x = 25 \times 0.71$
$x = 17.7$ m

The time taken for the ball to hit the turf is 0.71 s, and the horizontal distance travelled by the ball, for the team–mate to receive it is 17.7 m.

Example 2

A football is headed horizontally from a height of 2 metres into the opponent net, by an UNMARKED team-mate in splendid isolation. The football hits the net at approximately 5 metres from the point where it was headed.
Calculate the initial velocity of the ball.

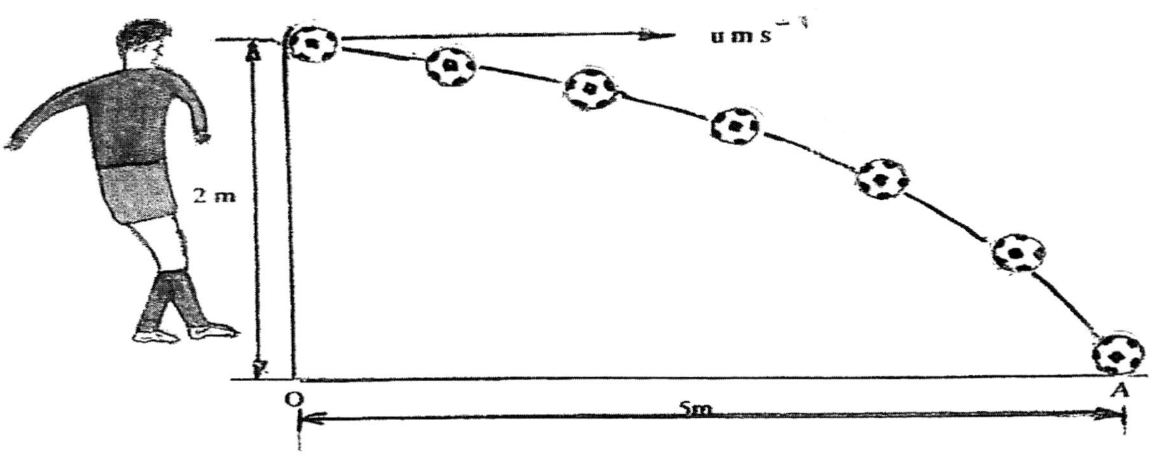

Fig. 15 - 5

Details of horizontal motion

$u = ?\text{ m s}^{-1}$

$s = 5$
$t = t$
$a = 0$

Details of vertical motion

$u = 0$
$s = 2$
$t = t$
$a = 0$

To find the time t for vertical motion

Use $s = ut + \frac{1}{2} at^2$

$2 = 0 + \frac{1}{2} (9.81) t^2$

$t^2 = \frac{2}{4.9}$

$t = \sqrt{\frac{2}{4.9}}$

$t = 0.64$ s

To find the initial velocity of the ball

Use distance = velocity x time

$5 = u \times 0.64$

$u = \frac{5}{0.64}$

$= 7.8 \text{ m s}^{-1}$

The initial velocity of the ball is 7.8 m s^{-1}

Headed Angle of Elevation above the Eye Horizontal

Example 1

A left back leaps, to head a ball over the top of the opponents to make a head clearance.

The initial velocity of the ball after impact is 10 m s^{-1}, and is headed at an angle of elevation of $\tan^{-1} \frac{5}{21}$ above the eye horizontal.

The ball lands 10 metres away at the feet of an UNMARKED team-mate in splendid isolation.

Calculate (a) the time for the ball to land at the feet of the UNMARKED team-mate.

(b) the height from the turf to which the left back has risen to make the headed clearance.

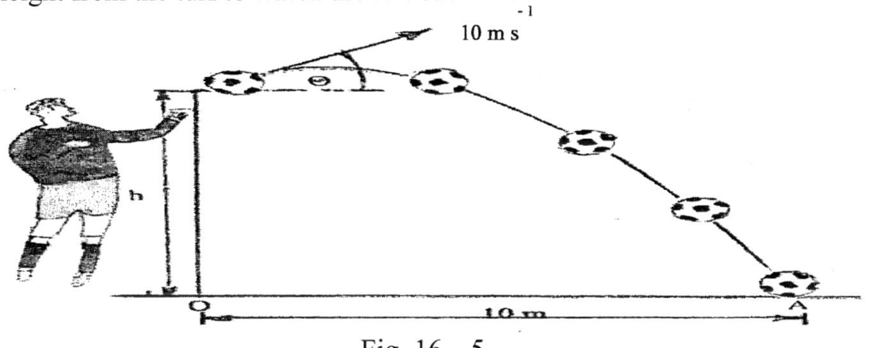

Fig. 16 – 5

The angle tan is given the sine, and cosine is found by using Pythagoras theorem, the sin $\theta = \frac{5}{21.5}$ and cos $\theta = \frac{21}{21.5}$

Details of horizontal motion

$u = 10 \cos\theta = 10 \cos\frac{21}{21.5} = 9.76 \text{ m s}^{-1}$

$s = 10$ m

$t = t$

$a = 0$

Details of vertical motion

$u = 10 \sin\theta = 10 \sin\frac{5}{21.5} = 2.32 \text{ m s}^{-1}$

$s = h$

$t = t$

$a = -9.81 \text{ m s}^{-2}$

To find the time the ball takes to reach the unmarked team-mate.

Use distance = velocity x time for horizontal motion.

$10 = 9.76\, t$

$t = \frac{10}{9.76}$

$t = 1$ s

To find the height of the leap from the turf of the left back

Use $s = ut + \frac{1}{2}at^2$ for vertical motion.

$h = -2.32\,(1) + \frac{1}{2}(9.81)\,1^2$

$h = -2.32 + 4.9$

$h = 2.5$ m

The time for the ball to reach the UNMARKED team-mate is 1 s.

The height of leap of the left back from the turf is 2.5 m.

In the same example in Fig. 16 – 5 if you convert $\tan^{-1}\frac{5}{21}$ to a decimal gives 0.2380 which is 13° from natural tangent tables cos 13° = 0.9744 and sin 13° = 0.2250

Substitution of these values into the formula will give a similar result.

Angle of Depression – Acute Angle – With The Eye Horizontal – Knock down Header

Example 1

A centre forward leaps to a height of 2 metres above the turf horizontal to head downwards an incoming cross from a winger.

The velocity of the ball is 20 m s^{-1} and the acute angle of depression is 35 degrees. Calculate the distance a team-mate will have to be in order to receive the ball.

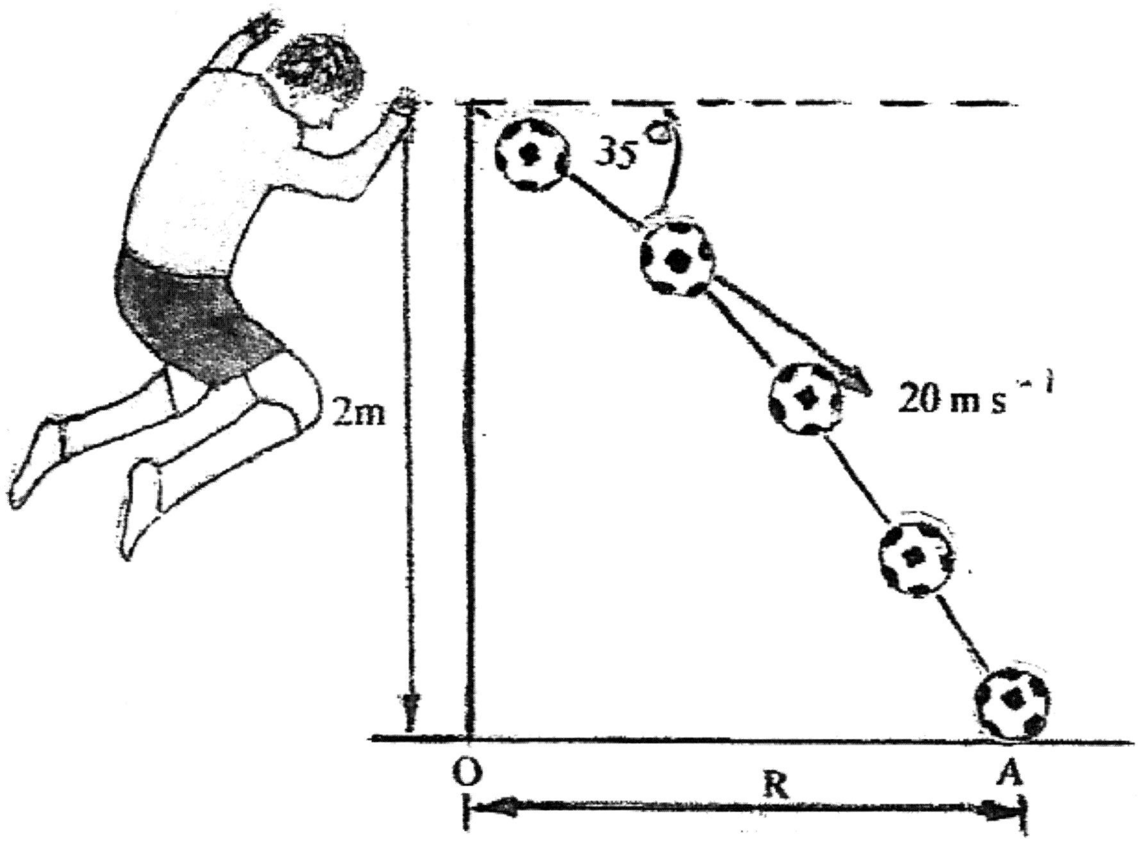

Fig. 17 - 5

Leap height of player y = 2 metres

Velocity of ball = $20\ m\ s^{-1}$

Acceleration due to g = $9.81\ m\ s^{-2}$

x =?

Using

Horizontal component $x = v\ t \cos 35^{o}$

Vertical component $y = -\ v\ t \sin 35^{o} - 0.57\ g\ t^{2}$

To calculate the time t the quadratic equation formula is used.

$$20\ t\ (-\ 0.57) - 0.57\ g\ t^{2} = -\ 2$$

$$4.9\ t^{2} + 10\ t - 2 = 0$$

$$t = \frac{-\ 10 \pm \sqrt{10 - 4(4.9)\text{-}2}}{2 \times 4.9}$$

$$t = \frac{-\ 10 \pm \sqrt{100 - 39.2}}{9.81}$$

$= \sqrt{139.2}$

$= \dfrac{11.7 - 10}{9.81}$

$= \dfrac{1.7}{9.81}$

$t = 0.17$ s

$x = v\,t \cos 35^{o}$

$= 20 \times 0.17 \times 0.819$

$= 2.78$ m or approx. 3m

The distance a team–mate will have to receive the ball is approximately 3 m.

Laws Of Motion – dynamic energy change - discovered by Sir Isaac Newton

Law 1

A ball continues in its state of rest or uniform motion in a straight line, unless acted upon by other forces. If a footballer starts a run from rest, he / she cannot instantly get up to speed, no matter how hard he / she tries, and this works in reverse, where the player once attains the speed, he / she cannot instantly stop. There must be a time interval for reaching a certain velocity, and to stop from that velocity.
When the brakes are applied to a forward moving car – the occupants tends to move forward – because they tend to maintain the original velocity possessed by the car.
These laws are very useful in dealing with ball motion and complete ball control by the players.

Law 2

The rate of change of momentum of a body is proportional to the force and takes place in the direction in which the force acts. This law has the same effect in producing motion, regardless of the state of motion or whether the force is alone or acting with other forces. This law involves mass and acceleration – keeping the force the same, and varying the mass, the acceleration varies.

Law 3

Action and reaction are always equal, and opposite.
If a rope is tied to a post, and a man / woman pulls the rope with a force of 100 N – the rope will resist to the extent of 100 N: according to Newton's third law, the reaction of the post is also 100 N.

Momentum

Momentum is defined as the quantity of motion in a body, and is measured by the product of its mass, and its velocity.

momentum = mass x velocity, and is a vector quantity with units of Ns

If a football collides with a player, the goal post or the goal bar, its velocity alters, and so does its momentum – Newton's second law.

Example 1

If a centre half weighs 75 kilograms, and moves with velocity of 2 m s^{-1}. Calculate the momentum of the centre half.
momentum = mass x velocity
= 75 x 2
momentum = 150 N

Example 2

If a football of weight 0.4 kg is kicked at a velocity of 30 m s^{-1}.
Calculate the momentum of the football.

momentum = mass x velocity
= 0.4 x 30
momentum = 12 N

Change in momentum is calculated by subtracting the initial momentum from the final momentum.

Work – Power – and Energy

Because a football / soccer game involves making an effort: this effort may take the form of running, change of pace, leaping, falling over, ball control, passing, possession - the defining moment in defence, and of the final ball: these factors and more concerns work, power, and energy.
For example, to use work, power and energy effectively and to conserve energy, team–mates must pull their weight equally to have an even distribution of work, power, and energy within the team: by not over-hitting or under-hitting a cross or a pass for a team–mate to have to expend unnecessary energy to get the ball.

A team–mate unmarked in splendid isolation, and his/her team-mate with the ball did not bother to look for him / her or two team-mates making runs into different striking positions, and the team-mate with the ball passes the ball to the team-mate in the worst striking position, and the chance is wasted – these are some of the instances where work, power, and energy are wasted and must be avoided.

Work

Work is defined as force x distance. If a midfield player moves a football / soccer ball with a certain velocity, and with a constant force of 10 units through a distance of 5 units – the midfield player has done a certain amount of work, the amount of work is equal to 10 x 5 units, which is the product of the force multiplied by the distance = 50 units. Gravity, and resistance, also will affect the amount of work done.
If the midfield player takes the path of high resistance or leaps above the turf, he / she has to do more work to cancel that resistance, if he / she takes the path of low resistance, he / she has to do less work to over-come that resistance.
The unit of work is the joule written as J.

Work against gravity
Example1.
A goalkeeper raises a football of mass 0.4 kg through a vertical height of 2.5 m. Calculate the work done against gravity by the goalkeeper.
Use work done = mass x gravity x distance
0.4 x 9.81 2.5 = 9.81 J

Power

Power is defined as work done per sec or the rate of working – and revolves around man, animal, and machinery etc, variation of the force and the direction also affects the power. The unit of power is the WATT- 1 joule per sec = 1 WATT.

Example 1 horizontal motion

The right winger runs down the flank with a velocity of 7 $m\ s^{-1}$. Resistance to motion, including running with the ball is 20 N. Calculate the power of the winger.

Power = force x velocity
= 20 x 7
= 140 W
= 0.14Kw

Example 2 horizontal motion

The left winger runs with the ball at his / her feet with a constant force of 2 N for 3 seconds, and covers a distance of 12 m. Calculate the work done, and the rate of working by the player.

Work done by winger = 2 x 12
= 24 J

rate of work by winger = $\frac{24}{3}$
= 8 W

Example 3 – vertical motion

Before a right back makes a long throw – he / she picks up the ball vertically with a constant velocity of 2.5 $m\ s^{-1}$. The mass of the ball is 0.4 kg. Calculate the work done, and the rate of working by the right back before he / she makes the throw.

Work done against gravity in one second = 0.4 x g x h
= 0.4 x 9.81 x 2.5
rate of working = 9.81 J
rate of working = 9.81 W

Energy

Chapter 1 on health and fitness gives some details of energy derived from food intake with an amount of calories. In this Chapter, the energy that will be discussed is stored mechanical energy – and this is divided into kinetic energy, and potential energy. Kinetic energy can be converted into potential energy, and vice versa. When a football is kicked vertically upwards the ball is given a certain amount of kinetic energy by the kicker, and this kinetic energy gives the ball motion. As the ball travels upwards, its kinetic energy is used up by the time it reaches its highest point of travel – due to the force of gravity. At this highest point the kinetic energy is converted into potential energy. As the ball falls back to the turf, it is accelerated by gravity or its own weight, and the potential energy is converted back into kinetic energy. At the moment of impact with the turf, all the potential energy will have been converted into kinetic energy.

Kinetic Energy

Kinetic energy is defined as the energy, which a body possess by virtue of its motion. A moving object possesses kinetic energy – for example, a football kicked towards the net of goal causes the net to bulge.

If the football has a mass m, moving with a velocity u, is gradually brought to rest, in a distance s, by constant force f, against it – the kinetic energy originally possessed by the ball is equal to the work done against f.

Using the equation $v^2 - u^2 = 2as$

$$\text{Work done} = \text{force} \times \text{distance}$$
$$= f\,s$$
$$\text{but } f = m\,a$$
$$f = \text{work done}$$
$$= m\,a\,s \ldots\ldots\ldots\ldots(1)$$
$$\text{Using } v^2 - u^2 = 2as \text{ when } u = 0$$
$$v^2 = 2as$$
$$a = \frac{v^2}{2s}$$

Substitute the value of a in equation (1)

$$\text{Work done} = \frac{1}{2} m v^2$$
$$\text{Kinetic energy} = \frac{1}{2} m v^2$$

Example 1

A football of mass 0.4 kg moving with a constant velocity of 30 $m\,s^{-1}$
Calculate the kinetic energy of the football.

$$\text{Kinetic energy} = \frac{1}{2} m v^2$$
$$= \frac{1}{2} \times 0.4 \times 30^2$$
$$= 180\text{ J}$$

The kinetic energy of the ball is 180 J

Thermodynamics is about energy – energy that is mathematically abstract and how it is transformed. The energy concerned with the internal state of a system is dependent on such parameters such as temperature, and pressure.
With respect to the air molecules within the ball – the internal energies represent the kinetic and potential energies of the molecules, and atomic particles that make up the system. Assume the wall of the ball to be perfectly insulated from its surroundings and there is no heat exchanged.
In a situation where a ball is kicked at the same time by two players – running into each other – the ball is sandwiched, and impacted by the feet of the two players which momentarily induces slight adiabatic compression, and expansion, a heating, and cooling process is carried out, and if, the process continues, internal changes within the ball cease to exist, and the system is said to be in a state of internal equilibrium.

If the pressure of a football is low, and when the ball is kicked deformation will last longer depending on how low the pressure is, how old the football is and the material the football is made of. If the pressure is very low deformation could even be permanent.
If the pressure is correct – kicking the ball continuously during the game will also cause the football to deform or the football's roundness is affected to some extent depending on the magnitude of the applied

force. In addition to these problems there are other natural forces, and air properties that cause the football to move in the air to varying degrees.
Good passing, moving and implementing the DEFINING MOMENT OF THE FINAL BALL depends on a ball that is correctly inflated, and well balanced.
The molecules of air within the football strike the wall at a point at an angle θ, and bounces off at an equal angle θ. The molecule loses no kinetic energy, and therefore its velocity is unchanged. Because of the geometry of the ball the molecules bounces continuously round the inside of the football.
The aimless motion of the air molecules within the football – its kinetic energy is temperature dependent: and is known as molecular thermal agitation: When a football is moving through the air its kinetic energy is greater than when the football is standing still – but the aimless motion, and temperature of the air molecules within the football remains unchanged.
The internal energy of air molecules is the kinetic energy caused by thermal movement, and depends on the number of atoms in the molecules of each individual gas. The gases are monatomic, diatomic, and have varying degrees of moment of inertia - rotational, and translational with variable degrees of freedom.

Potential Energy

Potential energy, is defined as the energy which a body possess by virtue of its position – examples of potential energy are a coiled spring or a car parked on the top of a hill – these possess potential energy, because it arises from its position, and not from its motion: if the spring or car, is set free from their position there will be motion. When an object of mass m kg is raised vertically upwards a distance h m, the work done by resisting gravity g is equal to the potential energy of the object. Potential energy is equal to mg h – and the unit for potential energy is the joules represented by J therefore P E = m g h.
Example 1 – A football of mass 0.4 kg is at a height of 10 m vertically above the turf. Calculate the potential energy of the ball.

$$
\begin{aligned}
PE &= m\,g\,h \\
&= 0.4 \times 9.81 \times 10 \\
&= 39.2\text{ J}
\end{aligned}
$$

As the ball descends it loses its potential energy.

HOOKE'S Law and Young's Modulus of Elasticity

A strain is proportional to the stress within the elastic limit – this is known as HOOKE'S LAW.
For a material when the stress is plotted against the strain will produce a straight line graph up to a particular point – beyond this point when more stress is added the straight line starts to curve – addition of more stress the material will reach its yield point, and eventually break.
The ratio of cross–sectional stress / longitudinal strain under tension or compression is called the YOUNG'S MODULUS OF ELASTICITY.

Law of Conservation of Energy

The law of conservation of energy states that in any system energy cannot be created or destroyed, although may change from one form to another.

Elastic Impact –

The calculations, where the ball is struck with various parts of the body, especially the head and feet, are based on Newton's law of restitution – for elastic impact, and impulse. To simplify the calculations, it is assumed that the ball is a perfectly elastic particle and the coefficient of restitution of 1 is used.

When a football is kicked, and strikes a surface, there is a moment of impact at this point in time the ball suffers some compression, and temporary change of shape. This moment of compression is followed by a moment in which the ball regains its shape, and its momentum or restitution.

The coefficient of elasticity is denoted by the letter e and is related to the ratio:

$$\frac{\text{Momentum after impact } v}{\text{Momentum before impact } u}$$

This is known as Newton's law of restitution

$$v = e\,u$$

A moving football possesses kinetic energy – a still football possesses no kinetic energy. To stop a moving football all its kinetic energy must be absorbed in some way: in order to do this – work must be done, and this work must be equal to the kinetic energy. For example, a goalkeeper makes a point blank save – first he / she has to cushion the ball then hold on to it.

Elastic Impulse – Collision with the goal post – pressure impulse

The force acting on an object for a short time is the product of the force and time - this is equal to the impulse.
When a force p is applied to a football of mass m for a time **t** its initial velocity changes from u to v. If the ball bounces back off the post, along the line of action of the force, the impulse is equal to the final momentum minus the initial momentum. The letter J is used to denote the impulse.

$$J = m\,v - (-\,m\,u)\ \text{N.}$$

An impulse J acting in a direction and making an angle θ is equal to an impulse, $J \cos \theta$ in a horizontal direction, and $J \sin \theta$ in a vertical direction are the changes of momentum in a horizontal, and vertical direction.

When the boot or head of a footballer, strikes a football, it is quite difficult to measure the magnitude of the force at any instant or the time during which the force acts, but it is possible to measure the change in momentum which the force causes, and hence the impulse.
As a matter of interest development of slow motion camera technology can make the measure of time during which the force acts quite real.

Impact and impulse are of significant importance, especially when a player heads a ball travelling at a high velocity. When the footballer heads the ball – the direction of the ball changes – and so does its momentum: the brain set in a protective fluid within the head absorbs a high percentage of kinetic energy – the shock waves taking the path of least resistance to the brain. These are so important when running with the ball.

If the force of the football exerted on the brain, is greater than the safety limit of the protective fluid around the brain: damage may occur. Another additional problem is a footballer, who runs in to head an incoming football at high velocity – here you have relative velocity: that is the velocity of the player moving forward, plus the velocity of the ball moving toward the player, so the brain absorbs an even greater amount of kinetic energy.
It is vital footballers know their limitations from a young age, and apply caution where necessary. Some players are better equipped to head a ball than others, because of varying bone thickness.

Over inflation of a football / soccer ball increases the impact on the head – because the coefficient of restitution becomes higher – the surface stiffness increases. Young people who play football / soccer should perfect practice heading with smaller and lighter balls before going on to the larger and heavier balls – find out their heading impact limitations.

When the ball is wet – its weight increases by a small amount. The forehead is the safest part of the head to head a ball at various angles. The neck muscles must be strong enough – prepared and ready to overcome the inertia of the ball at impact.

Intentional heading of the football / soccer ball is when the neck muscles are prepared and ready to head the ball, and to accept the impact. Accidental heading of the football / soccer ball is when the neck muscles are not prepared and ready to head the ball, and not ready to accept the impact – the player could feel the impact even more- it is at this moment that injury may occur.

In addition to linear kinetic energy when the football / soccer ball strikes the head of a player there is also kinetic friction from the spin of the ball at the moment of impact which increases the shock waves to the head.
Some caution and correct preparation are needed before heading an incoming football / soccer ball at a high velocity.

Example 1

A football of mass 0.45 kg when kicked on the turf toward the opponent goal hits the post at a velocity of $25\ m\ s^{-1}$. Assuming the coefficient of restitution is 1. Calculate (a) the velocity of the ball, as it bounces off the post. (b) the impulse exerted on the ball by the post.

(a) To calculate the velocity of the ball, as it bounces back off the post -
Use the law of restitution $v = e\ u$

$$v = 1 \times 25$$
$$= 25\ m\ s^{-1}$$

(b) To calculate the impulse exerted on the ball, as it bounces back off the post-
Use impulse $J = m\ v - (-\ m\ u)$

$$J = m\ v - m\ (-\ 25)$$
$$= 0.4\ (25 + 25)$$
$$= 20\ N$$

The bounce back velocity of the ball is $25\ m\ s^{-1}$
The impulse exerted on the ball by the post is 20 N

The momentum of the ball is changed – but the momentum of the post, which does not move is not changed.

Example 2

A right-winger makes a cross to a team-mate, who gets away from his marker in the opponent 18 yd box. The UNMARKED team-mate then head's the ball into the opponent net at $25\ m\ s^{-1}$. The mass of the ball is 0.45 kg, and its velocity before impact is $25\ m\ s^{-1}$.
Calculate the impulse given by the UNMARKED team–mate's head to the ball.

To calculate the impulse given by the player's head to the ball –
Use $J = m\,v - (-\,m\,u)$

The final momentum of the ball is 0.45×25 N
$= 11.25$ N
The initial momentum of the ball is $0.45\ (-\,25)$

$= 11.25$ N
$J = m\,v - (-\,m\,u)$
$= 11.25 - (-\,11.25)$
$= 22.5$ N

The impulse given by the UNMARKED team-mate to the ball is 22.5 N for a short time.

Example 1

A centre half of mass 75 kg runs in to head a ball at $7\ m\ s^{-1}$ collides with a centre forward of mass 70 kg running in to head the same ball at $5\ m\ s^{-1}$. The centre forward moves in the opposite direction after impact, at a velocity of $1.5\ m\ s^{-1}$.
Calculate the velocity of the centre half – assuming no external forces act during the collision.

Before impact

mass of centre half = 75 kg
velocity of centre half = $7\ m\ s^{-1}$

mass of centre forward = 70 kg
velocity of centre forward = $5\ m\ s^{-1}$

After impact

velocity of centre half = $u\ m\ s^{-1}$

velocity of centre forward = $1.5\ m\ s^{-1}$

The total momentum before impact = $75 \times 70 \times (-\,5)$ N
The total momentum after impact = $75\,u + 70 \times (1.5)$ N

$$525 - 350 = 75\,u + 105$$
$$175 = 75\,u + 105$$
$$175 - 105 = 75\,u$$
$$70 = 75\,u$$
$$u = \frac{70}{75}$$
$$= 0.9\ m\ s^{-1}$$

The velocity of the centre half is $0.9\ m\ s^{-1}$ in the same direction.

Example 2

A striker kicks a ball on the turf in a straight line, and the velocity of the ball is $20\ m\ s^{-1}$ – the striker made a mistake with his control angle – and instead of the ball going into the opponent net, the ball strikes the right hand post at an angle of 35 degrees to the post surface.
Calculate (a) the velocity of the football after impact.
(b) the angle of the football after impact.

(a)

Using - horizontal and vertical components before and after impact.

Before impact

$20 \sin 35^{o} = 20 \times 0.573 = 11.46$

$20 \cos 35^{o} = 20 \times 0.819 = 16.38$

At impact J = N

After impact the ball bounces off the post, and its velocity and direction changes.

Using $u = e\,v$

$u = 1 \times 11.46 = 11.46$

To find the velocity of the ball after impact use

v = square root of the sum of the squares of the horizontal components plus the vertical component.

$v = \sqrt{(11.46)^2 + (16.38)^2}$

$= \sqrt{131.3 + 268.3}$

$= \sqrt{399.6}$

$v = 19.9 \text{ m s}^{-1}$

(b) To calculate the angle made by the football after impact –

Use $\tan \theta = \dfrac{u}{20 \cos 35^{o}}$

$= \dfrac{11.46}{16.38}$

$= 0.699$

$\theta = 35^{o}$

If a coefficient of restitution of 0.8 is used for the football – the angle after impact will be different –

$8.0 \times 11.46 = 9.1$

$= \dfrac{9.1}{16.38}$

$\theta = 0.541$

$\theta = 28^{o}$

The velocity after impact will also change.

Inertia

Inertia is defined as the tendency of a body to resist the change of motion - keep its state of rest or uniform motion in a straight line – useful to the footballer where crossing, passing, heading and running with the ball: not to over-hit or under-hit the ball: needs slide rule accuracy.

Moment OF Inertia

The moment of inertia is in the kinetic energy of a rotating football – its angular momentum, and the momentum about the axis of the forces acting on it. Moment of inertia is derived from kinetic energy and angular velocity. Where the football is concerned, it is the spin of the ball or the kinetic rotational energy of the ball – especially for the bouncing ball, and for ball control: juggling where the spin of the ball is essential to lifting of the ball by the toe of the boot. The footballer has to attain a certain amount of spin of the ball with his toe before he can lift the ball unto his / her thigh, and then unto his / her head. Moment of inertia is also used for striking the curve path ball over – or around a wall of players – and for in - swinging corners.

Angular Velocity

Angular velocity is defined as the ratio of the change in angle by the change in time.
Other forms of measure are in degrees and radians. A radian is defined as the angle subtended at the centre of a circle by an arc equal to the radius of the circle.
If a point on a football / soccer ball makes 8 revolutions in 1 minute, then its angular velocity is 8 revs per minute.

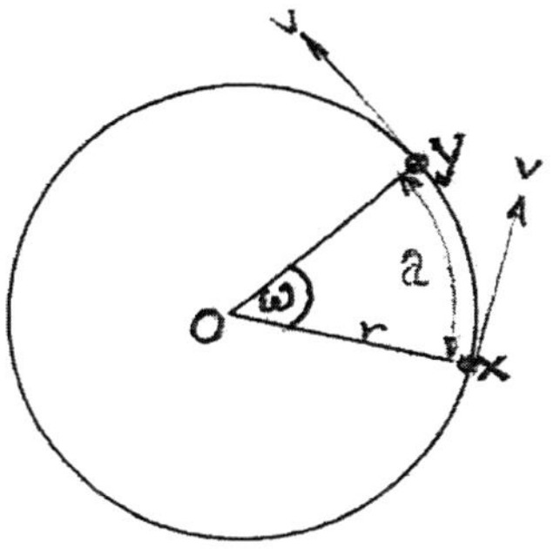

Fig. 18 – 5

Consider two points on a football – soccer ball. If point x travels from x to y the radius (r) ox travels through an angle θ, then the angular velocity ω (omega) about the centre o is by definition the change of the angle for every second.
Therefore if, t is the time for point x to travel to point y

$$= \frac{\theta}{t}$$

If the length of the arc x y is a then

$$\frac{a}{r} = \theta$$

Therefore $a = r\,\theta$

But t is the time taken to travel from x to y

Therefore $\frac{a}{t} = \frac{r\,\theta}{t}$

and $\frac{a}{t}$ = to the velocity v, and $\frac{\theta}{t}$ is the angular velocity

Therefore $v = r\,\omega$

Angular velocity is usually given in radians per second. It is the velocity of a point, which is rotating about a centre. The point as it moves plots a number of points to form a circle. A complete revolution is equal to 2 π or 6.2 radians – so if, the point makes one revolution in one second – the point would be travelling at 6.2 radians per second.

If a point P is on a football / soccer ball, and the ball rotates through 10 degrees – the corresponding distance moved by the point P would be -

$$\frac{10^{o}}{360} \times 2 \pi r$$

so the distance x travelled by the point P for any angle θ turned by the football / soccer ball is calculated by

$$x = \frac{\theta^{o}}{360} \times 2\pi r$$

(1) If a football / soccer ball of radius 12 cm turns through an angle of 25 degrees the point P on the circumference will move along the arc length x by –

$$x = \frac{25^{o}}{360} \times 2\pi r$$

$$x = \frac{25^{o}}{360} \times 2 \times 3.14 \times 12$$

$$x = 0.069 \times 2 \times 3.14 \times 12$$

$$x = 5.2 \text{ cm}$$

(2) To convert rev min^{-1} to rad min^{-1}

Convert 10 rev min^{-1} to rad min^{-1}

1 rev = 2π rad

10 rev = 10 x 2π rad min^{-1}

= 20π rad min^{-1}

and to convert rad s^{-1} to rev min^{-1}

2π rad = 1 rev

$$10 \text{ rads} = \frac{10}{2\pi} = \frac{5}{\pi} = \frac{5 \times 60}{\pi} = \frac{300}{\pi} \text{ rev min}^{-1}$$

A football / soccer ball when kicked at an angle of elevation for example – implementing the curve path strike the football develops a certain amount of spin or moment of inertia on its way to the goal – in this spin contains the angular velocity of the football.

Consider the leg of a player pivoted at the hip. If the player moves his / her leg back and forth you will notice that the foot follows the path of an arc, where the leg becomes the radius of the circle of which the arc is part of. If a player decides to strike a ball the foot velocity before impact can be calculated, if the radius, and the angle subtended from the centre to the arc points are known. The impact will be greater when the player accelerate before striking the ball – and the larger length and leg mass will also increase the impact even greater due to the linear and angular momentum.

(3) calculate the velocity in $m\,s^{-1}$ of a point on a spinning football / soccer ball of radius 12 cm with an angular velocity of (a) 25 $rad\,s^{-1}$ (b) 500 $rev\,min^{-1}$

(a)
Angular velocity = 25 $rad\,s^{-1}$
Radius of ball = 12 cm = $\frac{12}{100}$ m
To calculate the velocity use equation $v = r\,\omega$

$$v = \frac{12 \times 25}{100}$$

The velocity = 3 $m\,s^{-1}$

(b)
angular velocity = 500 $rev\,min^{-1}$
radius of ball = 12 cm = $\frac{12}{100}$ m

$$= 500 \times 2\,\pi \text{ rad min}$$
$$= \frac{500 \times 2\,\pi}{60} \text{ rad s}$$

To calculate the velocity use equation $v = r\,\omega$

$$v = \frac{12}{100} \times \frac{500 \times 2\pi}{60}$$
$$= 6.2\ m\,s^{-1}$$

The velocity = 6.2 $m\,s^{-1}$

Deflection - a good example of Newton's first law of motion

When a football is deflected its motion and direction changes - sometimes a footballer strikes a ball, hoping the ball will take the path of least resistance, then occasionally an opponent or team-mate gets in the path of the ball or the ball strikes the post or underneath the bar, and the ball is deflected into his / her own net or somewhere else: a good reason why some strikers head or shoot into the opponents crowded 18 yd / penalty area – the goalkeeper on the other hand, almost always cannot do anything about it; at times it works for you and other times against you – example of impact and impulse.

Cross Wind and Ball's – Change in Direction - Newton's first law of motion

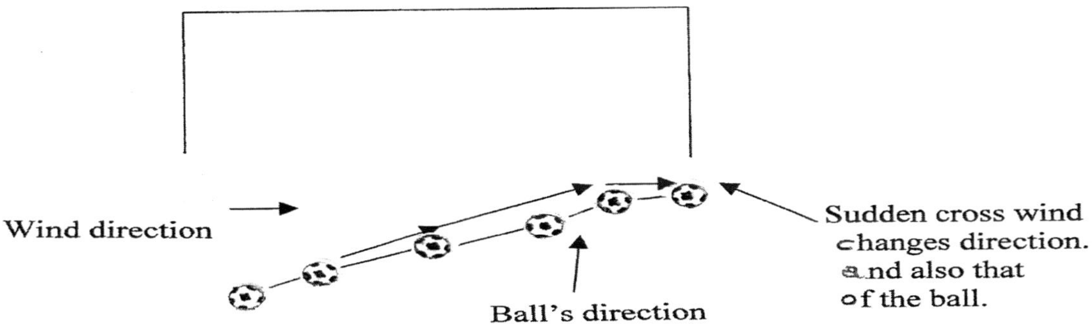

Fig. 19 - 5

Depending on the wind's sudden change in direction, and varying velocity – this could shift the ball off target after it has been struck – by a few centimetres or one or two metres: if it was intended to reach an UNMARKED team-mate or within an area near to one of the goalposts – in the horizontal plane and make it difficult for the player. The goalkeeper will also have some difficulty dealing with this type of ball in the vertical plane. The player will have to make allowances for wind changes and Newton's laws of motion.

Air Density – with Respect to the Ball

Air consists mainly of nitrogen, 78 % - oxygen, 21 % carbon dioxide, water vapour – the inert gases – hydrocarbons – sulphur compounds, plus traces of impurities.

The density of air from calculation or measurement is 1.25 kg / m. If the density of air increases drag resistance increases. When a football is kicked, reduced drag slows the football down at a slower rate, that is, the football will travel further. When a football is kicked – where the air is cool and dense, this cool dense air tend to slow the ball down, because the ball has to displace these denser air molecules out of its way.

Water vapour in air is a gas in air, and it is lighter than air, due to its molecular weight, compared to oxygen and nitrogen. Humid air is lighter than dry air, at the same temperature, and pressure – the football when kicked will travel faster, and further.

Density varies with pressure – temperature – humidity.

At low pressure air density is reduced and at high-pressure air density is increased.

When the air temperature rises, the air density decreases.

At high elevation, the air density is low.
At low elevation, the air density is high.

At low elevation – high pressure – and low temperature the air density is high.

Drag Coefficient – Friction Drag

With respect to a football, drag is the component of resultant force exerted by the wind on the ball parallel to the relative motion of the wind to the ball. Drag affects the football when the velocity and direction of the wind changes or does not change. For example, if a striker kicks the final ball toward the opponent goal, and the wind is blowing at a high velocity in the opposite direction of the ball – the wind is causing a certain amount of resistance to the ball, and the ball will slow down. If the football is struck in the same direction of the wind, the football will travel at a higher velocity – because there less friction drag – like it is easier for a boat to travel down a river, than it is to travel up a river. The velocity and the direction of the wind on the ball at other angles will also have a drag effect on the ball and this will cause the ball to – change its velocity and direction. Particle size, shape, and density increases or reduces the drag factor in a fluid.

The surface of the football, also plays an important role in increasing or decreasing drag – for example, if the football is not truly round or has uneven surface bumps – this will increase the drag on the ball – a smoother surface, reduces drag; modern cars, and aeroplanes are aerodynamically shaped to reduce drag to a minimum. The height of the grass, and the bumps on the surface of the pitch, also affect the velocity, and direction of the ball.

Drag coefficients are dependent upon Reynolds number at low or intermediate velocities - but independent at high velocities. Drag force is a function of elasticity, density, viscosity, and velocity of the wind, and a characteristic area concerned.
Drag equation –

$$\text{Drag in kg} = C_D\, p\, A\, \frac{V^2}{2}$$

C_D = Drag coefficient; dimensionless

p = the density of the fluid – wind; in kg / m^3

A = area on the ball relative to the motion of the fluid – wind in m^2

V = velocity of the wind with respect to the ball in $m\ s^{-1}$

Example 1

The diameter of a football is 24 centimetres, and is kicked by the striker with a velocity of 20 $m\ s^{-1}$. Assume normal temperature and pressure – calculate the resistance of the ball moving through the air – and the lift force. Use $C_D = 0.2$ for the drag coefficient and $C_L = 0.5$ for the lift coefficient.

$$\text{Use drag force} = C_D\, (\text{ air density } p\ )\, A\frac{V^2}{2}$$

Where $C_D = 0.2$
p = 1.25
A = 0.18 m^2 from Surface Area of a Sphere = $4\pi r^2$ and convert cm^2 to m^2
V = 20 $m\ s^{-1}$

$$= 0.2\ (1.25)\ (0.18)\ \frac{20^2}{2}$$

$$= 0.2\ (1.25)\ (0.18)\ 200$$

$$= 9\ N / m$$

The drag resistance of the ball moving through the air is 9N / m
For the lift force

$$\text{Use lift force } C_L = (\text{air density } p)\ A\frac{V^2}{2}$$

Where $C_L = 0.5$
p = 1.25
A = 0.18 m^2
V = 20 $m\ s^{-1}$

$$= 0.5\ (1.25)\ (0.18)\ \frac{20^2}{2}$$

$= 0.5\ (1.25)\ (0.18)\ 200$ The lift force = 22.5 N / m

Boundary Layer – Flat Surface

The boundary layer theory – was first presented by Prandtl. The boundary layer is the thin layer of air on a flat surface – consisting of thin layers of molecules.

Forces develop between the air and the flat surface in conjunction with the heat generated by friction drag during motion. At the flat surface the velocity of the air is zero, and changes to a free stream outside the boundary layer. As the air moves over the surface molecules of air stick to it : the layer of air molecules flowing above the first layer is slowed down by the surface molecules as they collide – consecutive layers of molecules are also slowed down as they move over the surface.
As the layers of molecules move away from the surface less collision takes place. A change in velocity in the stream wise direction causes a change in the other direction as well. The component of velocity perpendicular to the surface that moves the flow above it – is known as the lift drag. The horizontal component working parallel and opposite to the surface is known as the drag force.
Boundary layer over a flat surface continues to get larger in comparison to the boundary layer of a pipe where the radius of the pipe restricts the boundary layer. For a rough boundary the drag coefficient varies with roughness. For a low Reynolds number the flow is laminar – for high Reynolds number the flow is turbulent.

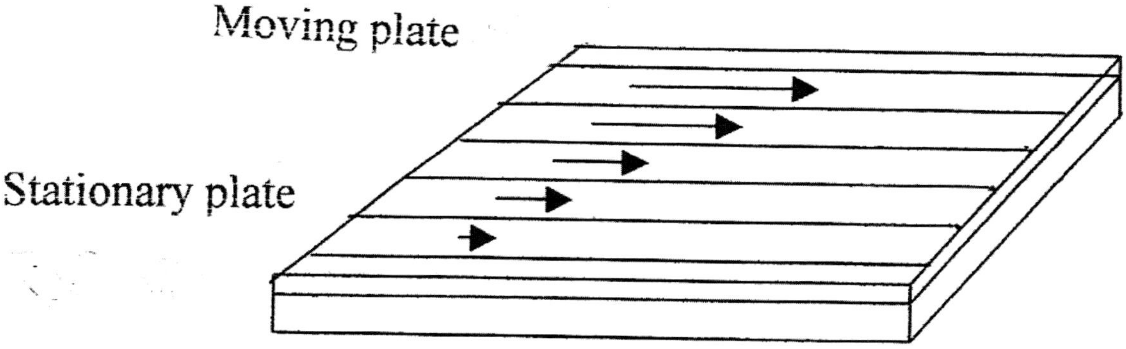

Laminar flow over a flat plate

Fig. 20 – 5

With a moving plate a layer of fluid moves with the plate – if the plate is stationary the layer of fluid is stationary, and the velocity of the fluid layers increase from the stationary to the moving plate with increasing velocities.

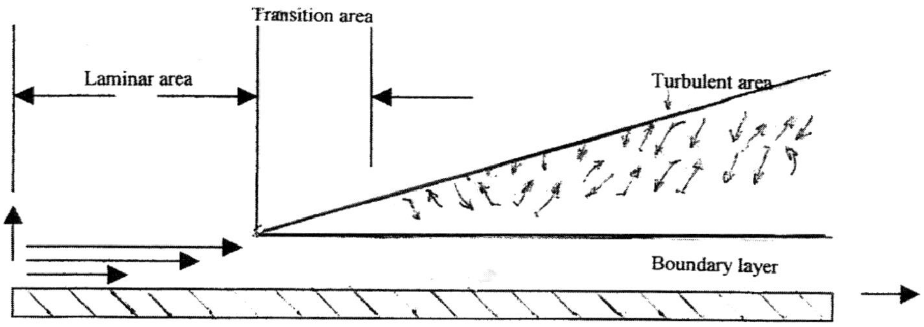

Laminar to Turbulent flow with Transition area

Fig. 21 – 5

Ball Motion and Direction In Relation To Player under Normal Conditions

When the velocity of the wind is high and the direction is changeable – the condition of the turf is soft or muddy; allowances will have to be made to compensate or deal with the situation the best you can.

With some understanding of basic fluid, and particle dynamics – the footballer is now in a better position to make the right split second decision on how to control the ball under most conditions with optimum efficiency. He will be able to understand, and reason as to why the ball behaves in certain ways, and the best way to deal with it.
As for the 4 dependent variables – ball control: passing: possession: and final ball – the footballer is now able to add that amount of care, finesse, skill, composure, and confidence to his / her play by Perfect Practice on the training ground, and implement that training on match days.

The various types of ball motion and direction commonly encountered in training, and on match days are as follows - these are good examples of Newton's laws of motion.

(1) The straight-line ball.
(2) The curved path ball.
(3) The dipping ball.
(4) The swerving ball.
(5) Ball falling freely – vertical, angled, before it strikes the turf, and the moment it strikes the turf.
(6) Ball strikes the turf, and starts to rise.
(7) Ball strikes the turf, rises, and then falls.
(8) Ball coming into player, at various heights, and angles – and off the turf.
(9) The low bouncing ball – straight line or otherwise.
(10) The smooth rolling ball on the turf straight line or otherwise.
(11) The deflected ball – deflected off the fixed goal post or bar, stationary or moving player: this is a hit or miss ball.
(12) The stationary ball.

The footballer should learn to identify the various types, Perfect Practice them on the training ground, and to know how to deal with all of them – that is complete control fluently, miss–control is not an option, and should be avoided as much as possible.

The most difficult balls to control are the ones that change velocity, and direction; some of these are as follows –

CURVATURE – SPACE CURVE – CURVE PATH or the BANANA KICK –
Small broken straight-line motion changing into curve path motion: the motion and direction of the ball is affected by a force that is perpendicular to this motion known as the lift or Magnus force, and this force opposes Newton's first law of motion to move the ball off its original straight line giving rise to small broken straight line motion - this causes a change in the direction of the ball, but the velocity of the ball does not change, and the ball takes a curve path.
When a football is kicked with the inside of the boot, the boot is wrapped around the ball, so to speak, to give it torque or turning effect to convert turn into spin or angular motion as the ball takes a curve path. It has rotational energy as well as translational energy.

When the inside of the right boot is used to strike the ball for a curve path strike – inward curling – the ball spins in an anti-clockwise direction as shown in Figs. 22 – 5, and 27 – 5.
Varying velocity of a football / soccer ball in a curve path is when there is a change in both the velocity and the direction of the ball caused by the force components in opposition with Newton's first and second laws of motion.

Out ward curling – similar in principle to inward curling except the outside of the boot is used to kick the ball, and the ball spins in a clock-wise direction.

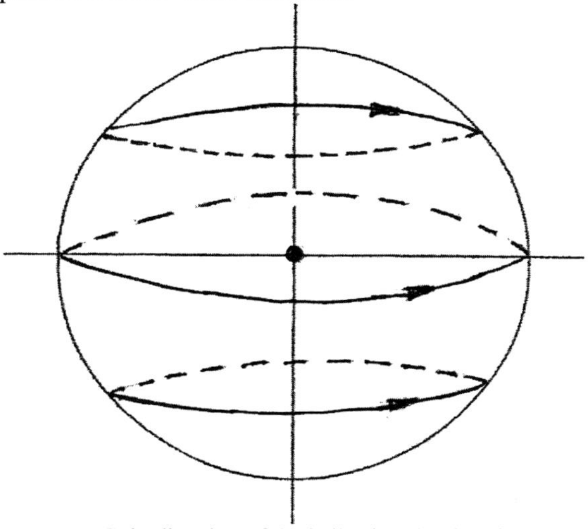

Spin direction of the ball using the right boot

Fig. 22 – 5

The space curve or curve path ball is a hit or miss strike for any striker, even the best player who can produce an excellent strike to score at times – cannot score every time he / she gets the chance: because of the vast number of dynamic and psychological factors to get right before the strike is taken – for example – weather conditions – the correct impact applied to the ball at the correct characteristic point on the ball – the correct centre of gravity of the kicker in relation to the correct characteristic point on the ball – placement of the opponent wall in relation to the goalkeeper – crowd noises, and the emotion of the kicker at the moment of impact. Plenty of Perfect Practice must be carried out in training to obtain a fairly good goal – scoring rate from this type of strike.

The energy and component forces responsible for the curve path ball are the correct kinetic energy at impact of the boot's correct characteristic point, on the correct characteristic point of the ball to give the necessary torque or turning effect to turn the ball into spin – drag and lift forces to change the straight-line or rectilinear motion into tiny broken line curvature, curvilinear or curve path motion.

Fig 23 – 5 shows when a spinning football is in flight the air moves quicker on one side, and slower on the other side – this causes a difference in pressure, and this pressure difference help to move the ball of its straight line. When a football / soccer ball is moving in a curve path, it is changing its direction all the time – this continuous change in direction, is caused by a force known as the lift force - Magnus force, in opposition with Newton's first law of motion.

When a football / soccer ball is moving through the air in the vertical plane – there are two forces and a pressure difference responsible for changing the ball's direction.

(1) The drag force, which acts in the opposite direction in which the football is moving.
(2) The lift or Magnus force which acts upwards, and in opposition to Newton's first law of motion, which is tends to keep a straight-line motion is responsible for helping the football to take the curved path.

During laminar flow as the air flows over the football there is a quick transition of the boundary layer of air molecules, the airflow spends less time on the surface of the ball – quick transition produces high drag. But as the airflow becomes turbulent, the boundary layer of air molecules sticks to the surface of the football for a longer time – slow transition produces small drag, Fig 23 – 5.

Turbulence happens when smooth flowing laminar flow becomes rough and haphazard. There is a critical Reynolds number where laminar flow becomes rough, and turbulence occurs. When the air velocity increases laminar flow will be in action, until a critical Reynolds number is attained, at which point the turbulence occurs. Increasing Reynolds number increases velocity – this increases the kinetic energy of the flowing air, and also generates sound waves. The critical Reynolds number corresponds to the transition from laminar to turbulent flow as the velocity is increased.

The surface of the football / soccer ball affects the Reynolds number – footballs with high surface roughness – increases drag friction.

When the strike is taken the centre of gravity of the kicker must be correct – the incorrect centre of gravity of the kicker will lift the ball too high or too low depending on the amount of lean back or lean forward that is used by the kicker, and a bad wall to keeper set up Fig. 24 – 5 or a good wall to keeper set up Fig. 25 – 5. The spin of the ball is caused by the kinetic friction between the boot and the correct characteristic point on the football that is a distance off the centre of gravity of the ball. An increase in the kinetic friction between the ball and the boot will cause the ball to gain more spin. There is an optimum position with respect to the correct characteristic points on the boot to the ball for the player to strike the ball in order to get maximum spin, Figs 26 – 5 & 27 – 5 too far, from the characteristic point and the ball will not spin or the spin will be a small amount. Depending on the impact, the average spin of a football / soccer ball in a curve path trajectory is approximately 8 to10 revolutions per second. If you can make the air flow turbulent on the surface of the ball by giving it a greater impact the drag force will stay small, and the ball will move through the air quicker.

With regards to weather conditions on a dry day the ball will gain more spin when struck at the correct characteristic point – and with the kicker's correct centre of gravity: because at impact of the boot to the football the kinetic friction gives the football a high percentage of torque or turning effect which causes the football to turn, and converts this turn into spin. The friction is greater due to the dryness of the boot and football when in contact – there is a greater grip between the boot and the football – and less slip – on a humid day the velocity of the ball tends to increase.

On a wet day there is a film of water between the wet boot, and the wet ball, this film reduces the kinetic friction between the boot and the football – and the grip between the boot and the football is reduced: the slip is increased to produce more slide, and this in turn produces less torque or turning effect, so the football turns less, hence less spin.

Boundary Layer – Drag on a Football / Soccer Ball

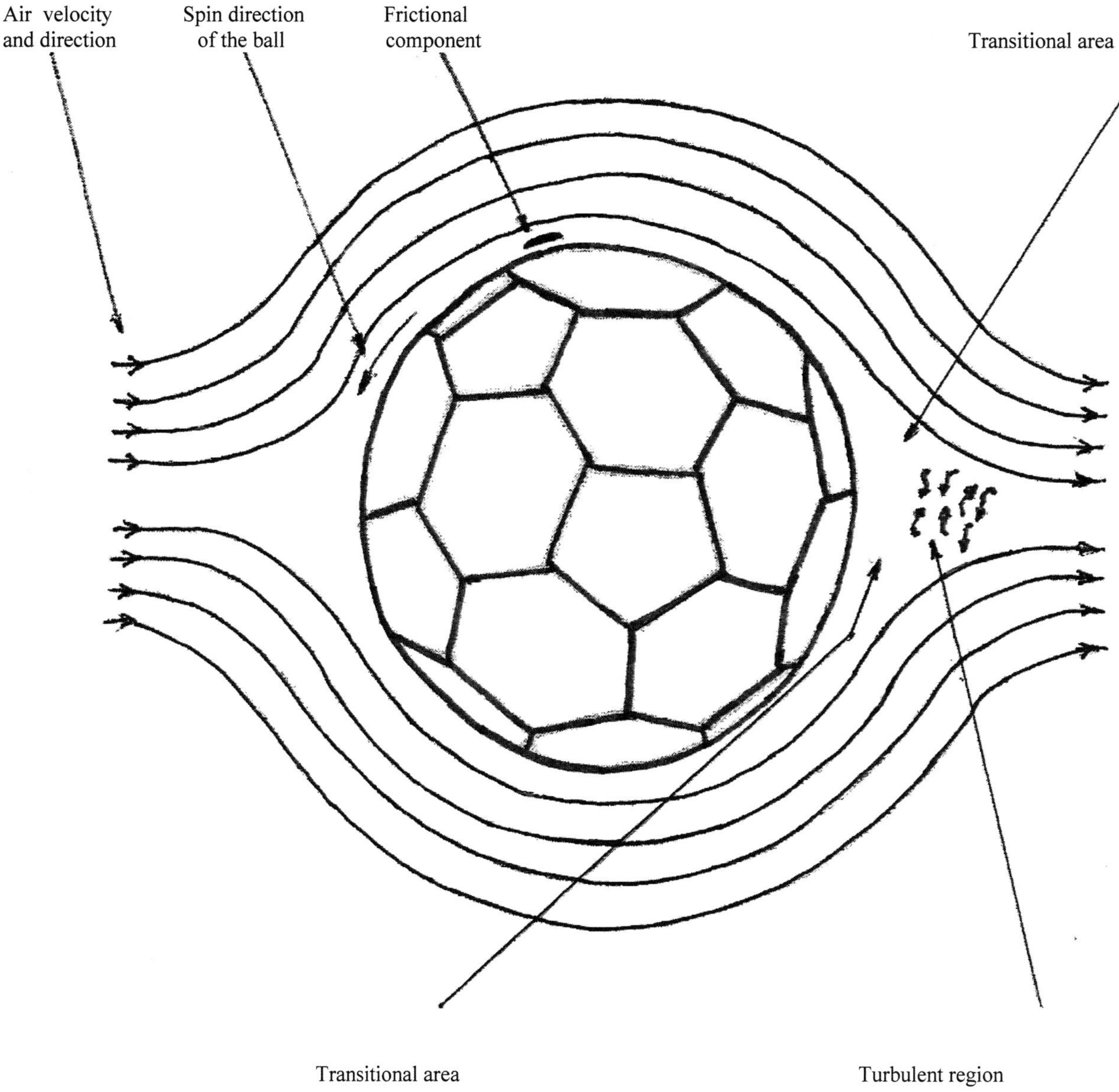

Fig. 23 – 5

Curve Path Ball – Bad Defence Set Up By the Opponent

Fig. 24 – 5 the keeper's position is good, in relation to the wall, but the wall is too far from the kicker – giving the kicker too much space to make the necessary adjustments required to implement the DEFINING MOMENT OF THE FINAL BALL for the curve path ball – the keeper is unable to get to the ball before it enters the net.

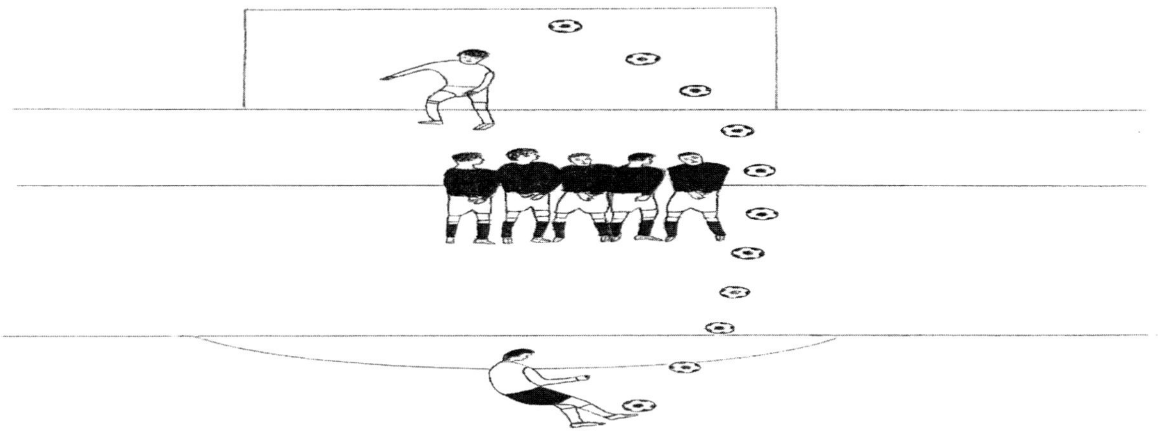

Fig. 24 – 5

Curve Path Ball – Good Defence Set Up By the Opponent

Fig. 25 – 5 the keeper's position on his / her line and in relation to the wall is good – the distance of the wall from the ball is good – this set up makes it quite difficult for the kicker to make the necessary adjustments to implement the DIFINING MOMENT OF THE FINAL BALL for the curve path ball – the keeper's acceleration, and leap are good enough to get to the ball, and tip it over the bar.

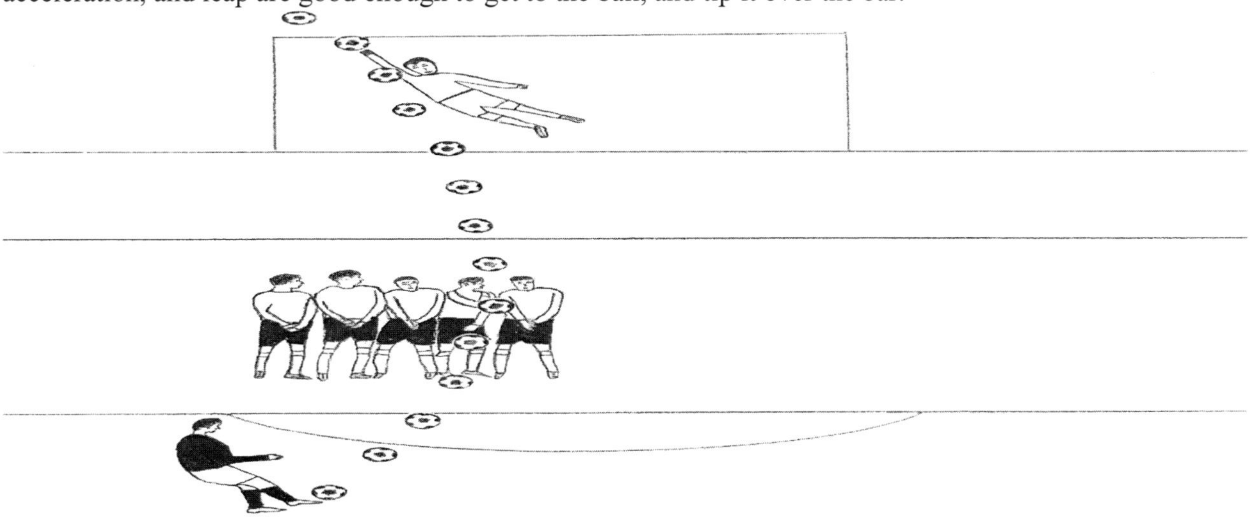

Fig.25 – 5

Towards the end of its journey, the football follows a curve path trajectory – it loses some kinetic energy and slows down – but the curve deviates and becomes larger. When the velocity of the football falls to a level where it entered the laminar flow region, this causes an increase in the drag on the football which in turn cause it to slow down even further – then the Magnus or lift force bends the ball into the goal while still opposing Newton's first law of motion, the drag coefficient increases and this causes the lift force to become larger, and the football curvature greater. On average it takes about 1 second from start to finish for this process to complete, depending on the distance from goal, and impact of the strike.

Characteristic Points on the Football / Soccer Ball for Space Curve or Curve Path Motion

Centre of gravity of ball.

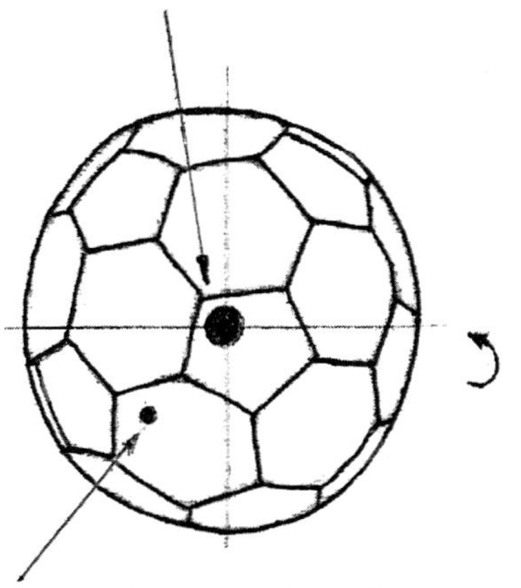

Characteristic point on ball – to produce turn into spin from the correct characteristic point on the boot – with respect to the kicker's centre of gravity.

Fig 26 - 5

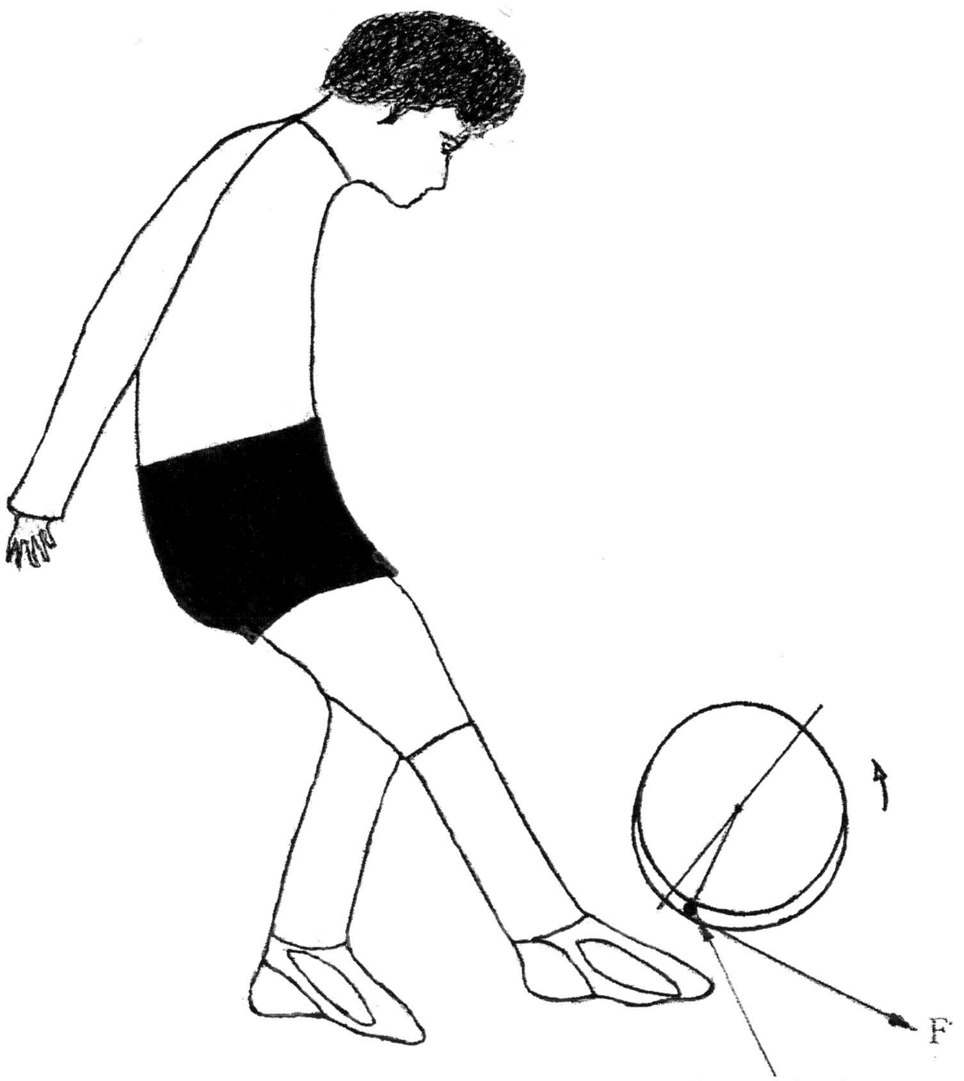

Fig 27 – 5

Imagine for a curve path strike the area containing the characteristic point on the ball, is a thin ring sliced off, the correct impact from the correct characteristic point on the right boot, to the correct characteristic point on the ball gives the ball a certain amount of torque or turning effect – like placing a spanner on a nut and turning it – except with the ball the turn is converted into spin very quickly, almost instantaneously. Inward curling the ball spins in an anti-clockwise direction – moments are positive. Outward curling the ball spins in a clockwise direction – moments are negative.

Dipping Ball

When a football is kicked toward goal, sometimes the ball dips under the bar – just before the bar or as it passes over the bar or the keeper on its flight toward goal the ball possesses kinetic energy and linear momentum: depending on the magnitude of the force applied to the ball – the ball travels a certain distance, and then it start to lose its kinetic energy and linear momentum: and the ball dips. If the ball is allowed to continue its flight it will eventually lose all of its kinetic energy and linear momentum, and the ball will start to fall to the turf: at the moment the ball strikes the turf – the ball loses its potential energy. When the ball eventually comes to rest, it will have lost all of its kinetic energy, linear momentum and inertia.

Swerving Ball

When a player kicks a football and it travels at a high velocity – it sometimes swerves as it approaches its target – this is due to a combination of varying air properties such as density, humidity, ambient temperature and pressure: air velocity and the direction – the air resistance or drag force on the ball. The ball is tending to take the path of least resistance through the air as it travels on its flight – that is – swerving around the lighter air molecules, especially on a humid day.

Falling and Rising Ball

These are difficult balls to control for making a cross, pass or final ball. The player will have to work out in a split second, whether the ball is falling or rising before he / she can control it, in order to strike it correctly. If the ball is rising, and the player tries to strike the ball, it will follow an upward path, because the ball will tend to maintain its original velocity, direction, and kinetic energy it originally possessed – Newton's first law of motion – a reason on many occasions rising ball struck towards the goal almost always goes over the bar, made worse by the player leaning backwards too much – this alters the player's centre of gravity, and the player gets underneath the ball, and cause the ball to lift even higher. The player should reduce the rise of the ball by getting on top off it, so that he / she can have better control to get the line of action of the force correct before striking the ball.

The falling ball is easier to control, because it tends to maintain its downward velocity, direction and kinetic energy, before it strikes the turf. A falling ball when struck with an effort to keep it low will follow a low path, and the player will have better control to strike the ball more accurately.

Players should pay attention to identifying, and dealing with rising and falling balls, and treat them with respect, particularly when the ball is required to be kept low - example when implementing the DEFINING MOMENT OF THE FINAL BALL.

Dynamic Friction – Rolling – Bouncing – Sliding Ball

When a football rolls on a smooth turf, the point of the ball in contact with the turf at any point in time is instantaneously at rest. The forces at the point of contact with the surface do no work, and hence the change in kinetic energy of the ball may be equated to the work done by other forces acting on the ball. When the football strikes another player it tends to maintain its linear velocity, but because it is rotating, the rotational energy changes the football's direction due to its impact angle.

As the football rolls, it has inertia in its translational and rotational linear motion. When a football moves on the turf a frictional force is exerted at the turf between the ball, and the turf – this frictional force is called the dynamic frictional force. When a body is in contact with the surface of another body, there is some resistance, which is known as friction.

There are two types of friction –

(a) Rolling friction
(b) Sliding friction

(a) Rolling friction is when an object such as a football rolls on the turf, and occurs mainly between hard surfaces.
(b) Sliding friction occurs between soft, hard surfaces and with a cylindrical surface contact with a surface is along a line: with a football contact with the turf is at a point - so long as the surface at the point of contact is hard.

Sliding friction is greater than rolling friction.

Lubricating or polishing a surface reduces friction. Friction increases with the roughness of surfaces, and is greatest at the start of motion. When a football is kicked at about one metre above the turf from outside the opponent 18 yd / penalty area, and bounces off the turf a few metres in front the keeper at a certain velocity: it also slides – as this happens sometimes the velocity of the ball increases, and sometimes the velocity decreases. This dynamic energy change in velocity is dependent on the condition of the turf – whether it is dry, wet, hard or soft and the forward or backward spin of the ball, Fig 4 – 3.

The reason the football accelerates from the first bounce, and slide motion at the point it makes contact with the hard turf is – when the football bounces, and slides, it possesses kinetic energy and is accompanied by kinetic or sliding friction. At the moment of impact of the football with the turf: the kinetic or sliding friction is greatest at the beginning of motion, and becomes zero as the football leaves the turf on the rise – at the same time a minute amount kinetic energy which the ball possesses is absorbed by the turf, and a vast amount is transferred back to the ball – because the football is an elastic particle, this kinetic energy gained by the football from the bounce causes the ball to accelerate depending on the forward, backward or no spin of the ball at contact with the turf. Forward spin of a ball propels it in a forward direction with increased acceleration – backward spin propels it in a backward direction with decreased acceleration at contact. No spin the ball will slide during the bounce.

On a soft turf surface the football strikes the surface, and deforms it, and there is more friction – the ball becomes stuck momentarily, and the increase in velocity will be less than that of a hard turf surface. Sometimes the turf surface may be hard, but slight rain or watering have wetted the surface – not to cause deformation of the surface, but to make it slippery: this would reduce friction, increase the velocity of the football, and cause it to accelerate – like walking on ice: you are suddenly on a skid, and your velocity increases.

A first bounce football is a difficult ball for the keeper to hold on to, because he / she has the problem of working out its change in velocity – after the bounce and slide of the football as it approaches the keeper especially if struck fiercely from just outside the opponent 18 yd box, the same applies to making an on the turf pass to an UNMARKED team-mate in splendid isolation, more control effort by the team-mate is required to control the ball.

Expect the Occasional Unexpected – The Goalkeeper

Low bounce and slide of ball – some goalkeepers may spill the ball due to its increase in velocity so they must be aware of this change in velocity of the ball: when the ball is coming in on the turf towards the keeper – he / she must get down quickly, get his / her body down on the turf, and behind the ball – and hold on to it. The downward velocity of the keeper must be such that his / her body is on the turf a split second before the ball reaches him / her. In this way the keeper does not leave any gaps for the ball to pass through. Expect the extra velocity of the ball when it bounces, and slides – and be prepared for it.

If the ball bounces once in front of the keeper, a few feet above the turf – the keeper must get his / her body behind the ball, and cushion it, to absorb the extra kinetic energy of the ball, gained by the bounce, and slide, and to hold on to it. If the goalkeeper happens to spill a shot from the opponent – this is where quick reaction and response from defending team - mates comes in to safely, and decisively clear the ball, away from dangerous areas or start a new move. Good backing up by defending team-mates is a must.

Chapter 6

The
Four Dependent Variables

Before players can defend or attack – four departments of play must undergo perfect practice over a number of weeks or months in order to reach optimum standard – once the standard is reached: it must be maintained.
The four dependent variables are some of the tools absolutely necessary for playing good exciting free flowing football / soccer, the DRIVE MECHANISM for defence and attack.
The four dependent variables are interconnected and are as follows -

(1) Ball Control (complete)
(2) Passing and Crossing
(3) Possession
(4) Final Ball – the DEFINING MOMENT OF THE FINAL BALL

Newton's first law of motion is interwoven into all four variables. All four variables are interwoven into each other: one depends on the other: one cannot do without the other – and are played in the horizontal and vertical planes – that is, 80% to 90% on the turf, and 10% to 20% in the air.

Ball Control and Newton's First Law

Perfect Practice - control of a ball under any condition. Make and receive slide rule crosses and passes, under any condition, with chest, head or feet – in conjunction with Newton's first law of motion.
At the moment of contact with the ball, the first touch – for that split second, the ball becomes an extended part of the player's chest, head or feet: it is at this moment of contact, that extra effort in control and direction must be applied to strike, the ball to its destination – requires COMPLETE BALL CONTROL.
Bad ball control could lose you possession, and give the opponent a chance to score.
Bad ball control is not an option.
Brain to chest, boot and head co-ordination – lock onto target – transfer thought from brain to chest, head or boot – LINE OF ACTION OF THE FORCE to the ball, then to the target.

Pick a target – take a ball in one hand, and throw it at the target: see how many times, you can hit the target or get near it. Try throwing the ball at the target without concentration – and then with concentration – check for improvement.

Using the ball, try it with chest, head, and feet on the real targets, such as the goal-mouth, and other team–mates. It takes time and Perfect Practice to get the line of action of the force right.

THE FIRST TOUCH OR THE MOMENT OF CONTACT IS THE KEY – This determines whether the player could control with accuracy – or little or no control.

Try sudden acceleration for a few seconds: then sudden retardation – and then sudden change of direction – without losing the ball. Then try it with opponents in pursuit – without losing the ball. Apply Newton's first law of motion.

Ball control is about the correct centre of gravity of the player's body in relation to controlling the ball with the chest, feet or head – the correct strike angles – cushioning the kinetic energy of the ball during impact, and application of Newton's first law of motion.

To control and trap a falling ball – control a rising ball – shield the ball from opponents – to make a one touch slide rule pass to an UNMARKED team-mate in splendid isolation.
To control various types of balls under varying velocity, direction, and conditions – see ball motion Chapter 5. When the ball is bouncing, and sliding on a dry day – on a wet day – and on a windy day.
Flicking the ball upwards - using the toe to juggle with both feet or to volley past the opponent keeper on a wet, dry or windy day.
Ball control under little or no pressure with time and complete space: ball control under a lot of pressure with two or three opponents surrounding you – not much time or complete space.
Ball control is about controlling the ball with precision during a head or foot strike. A good way to control a falling ball or a ball coming in at chest height, is to use the chest, because of its large surface area and cushioning property, Fig 1 – 10 Chapter 10, and ball control is to control the ball, so that you make the forces of nature work for you rather than against you.

Characteristic Points on the Boot

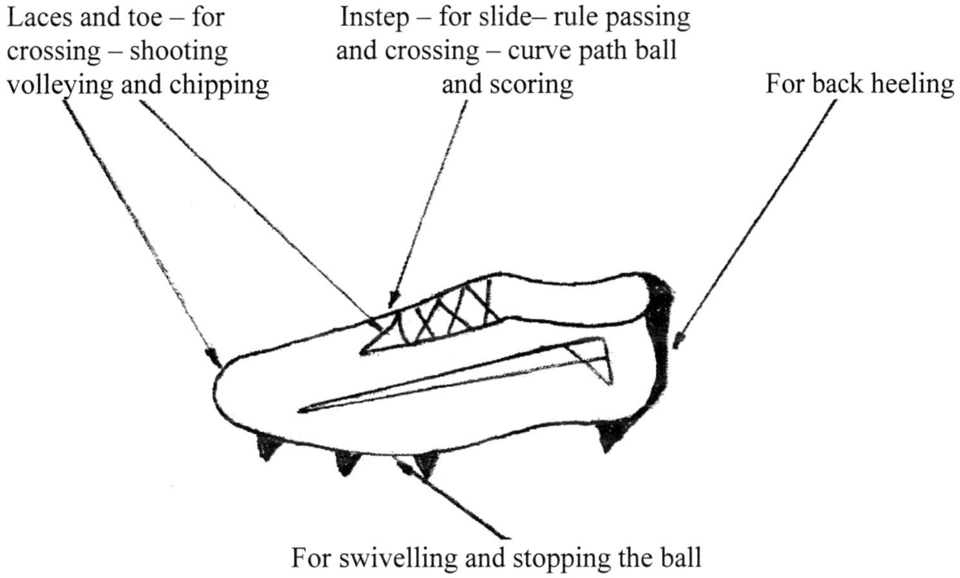

Fig 1 – 6

The main purposes of the correct football / soccer footwear for training and playing are for safety, and to prevent serious injuries to players and opponents. The players must be able to run efficiently with and without the ball – for good ball control, and be able to strike the ball accurately at the respective characteristic points. The footwear must be light – strong – comfortable and to cushion the impact of striking the ball – and from strong tackles.

Characteristic Points On The Ball

Striking position of the football with respect to the kicker's centre of gravity - the centre of gravity of the body must be altered for various striking positions.

Within the strike angle is the line of action of the force – in the horizontal and vertical planes.

For keeping the ball low
and within the 7 degrees,
acute angle of elevation strike -
on the turf strike surface to air

Rising off the turf –
top half of ball strike to keep it down,
centre of gravity, and posture must be correct –
to get on top of the ball – vertical plane

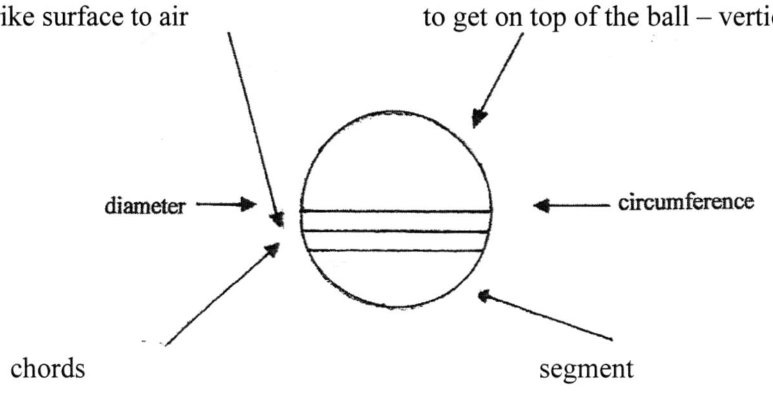

Fig. 2 – 6

Within the diameter, and
bottom chords – for on the
turf strike to keep the ball
down – horizontal plane

Bottom segment helps
to give the ball lift for
over the top cross or
pass – curve path ball -
vertical plane

For example – if a player receives a ball to implement the DEFINING MOMENT OF THE FINAL BALL – but the ball is rising, and spinning – what reaction and response the player must make to deal with this type of ball? The player must reduce the spin of the ball or its rotational energy as well as its upward velocity. Apply Newton's first law of motion.

Characteristic Points on the Football / Soccer Ball for Space Curve or Curve Path Motion – using the right boot

Centre of gravity on ball

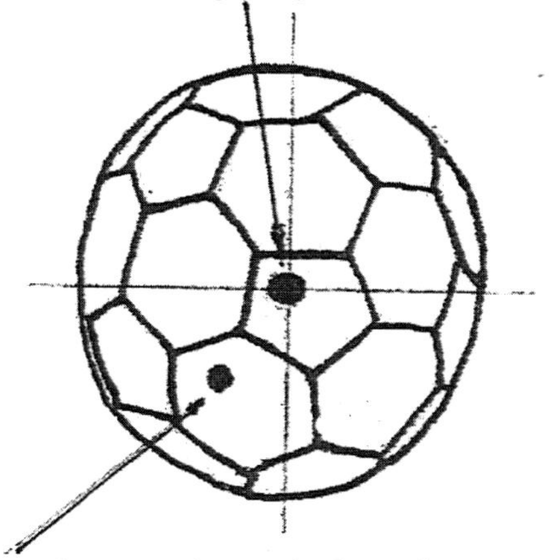

Characteristic point on ball – to produce turn into spin from the correct characteristic point on the boot – with respect to the kicker's centre of gravity –
Using the inside of the right boot – inward curling – the ball spins in an anti-clockwise direction.
Using the outside of the right boot – outward curling - the ball spins in a clockwise direction.

Fig. 3 – 6

Characteristic Points on the Football / Soccer ball for Space Curve or Curve Path Motion – using the left boot

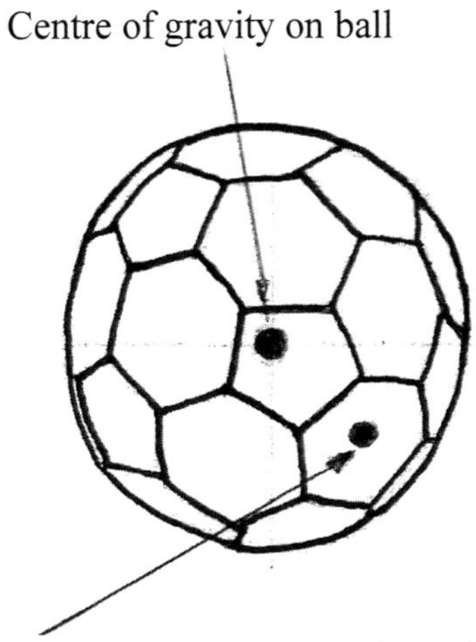

Characteristic point on ball – to produce turn into spin from the correct characteristic point on the boot – with respect to the kicker's centre of gravity.
Using the inside of the left boot – inward curling – the ball spins in a clockwise direction.
Using the outside of the left boot – outward curling – the ball spins in an anti-clockwise direction.

Fig. 4 - 6

Football / Soccer Ball Specification

Shape................Spherical
Diameter.............24 cm – approx.
Circumference......72 cm – approx.
Material...............Leather 2
Pressure............ 700 to 1000 gm cm – approx.
Weight...............410 to 450 gm

THE LINES OF ACTION OF THE FORCE IN RELATION TO THE INTENDED TARGET

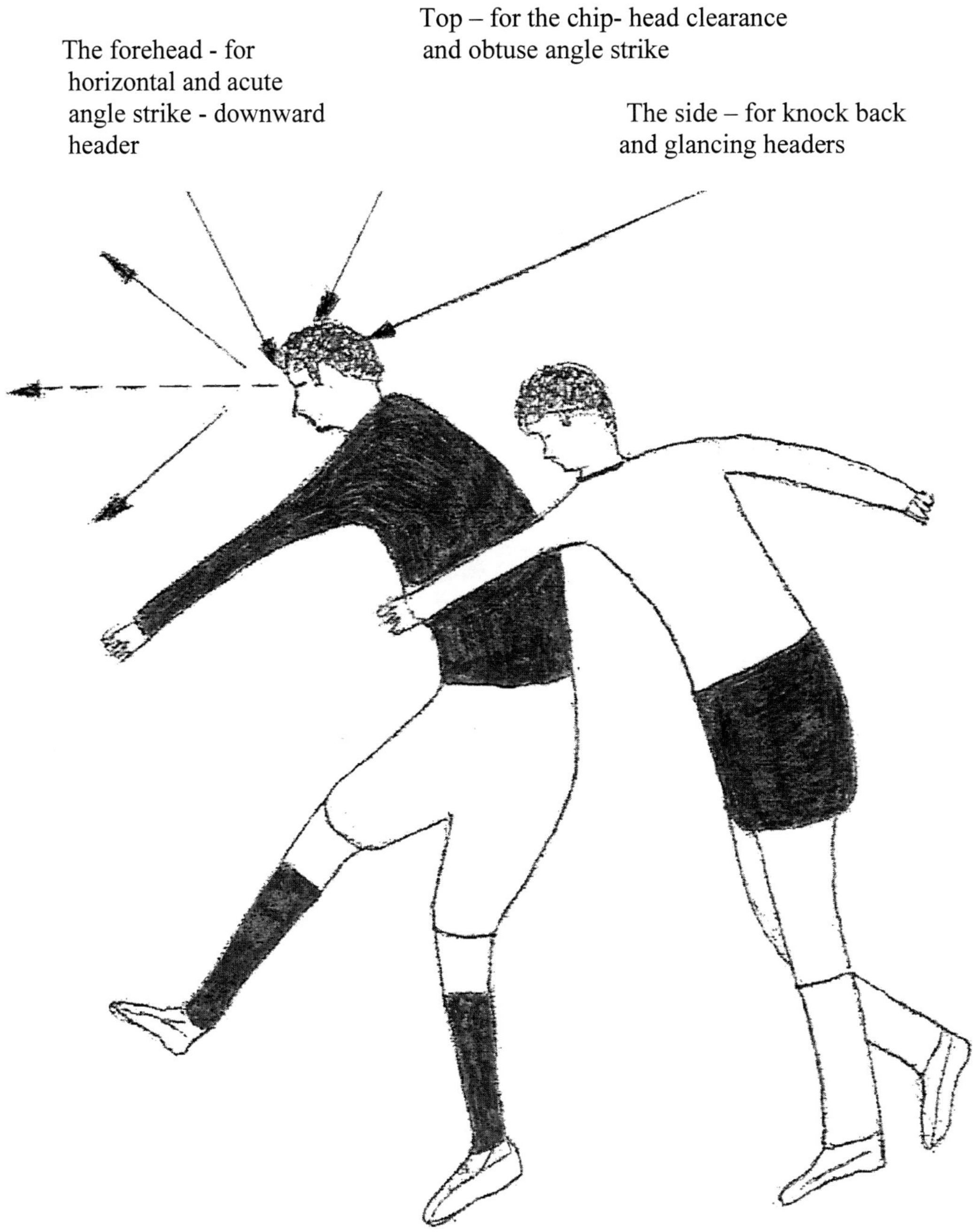

Characteristic Points on the Head Fig. 5 – 6

Angles for Turning Opponents

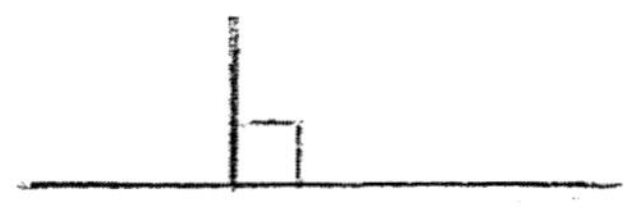

(a)

A quarter turn of 90 degrees in the horizontal plane, for passing and the DEFINING MOMENT OF THE FINAL BALL.

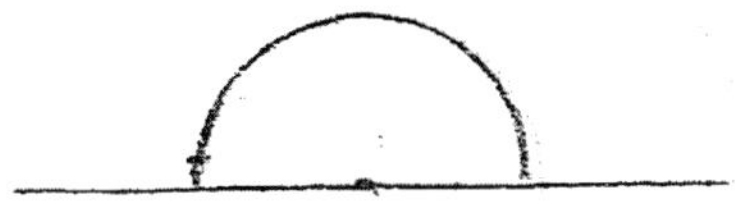

(b)

A half turn of 180 degrees in the horizontal plane, for passing and the DEFINING MOMENT OF THE FINAL BALL.

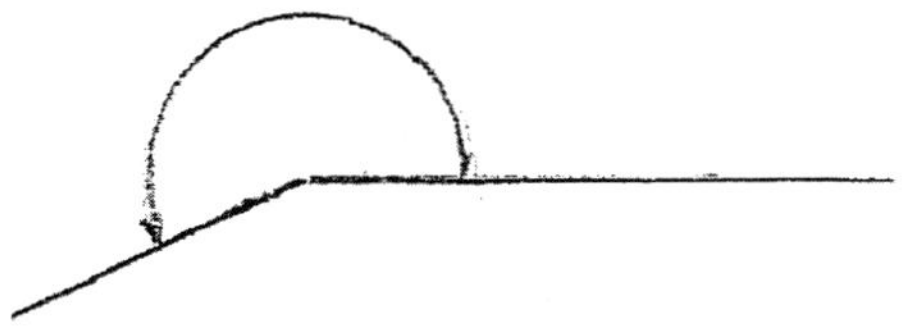

(C)

A reflex angle turn of more than 180 degrees – but less than 360 degrees – for passing and the DEFINING MOMENT OF THE FINAL BALL.

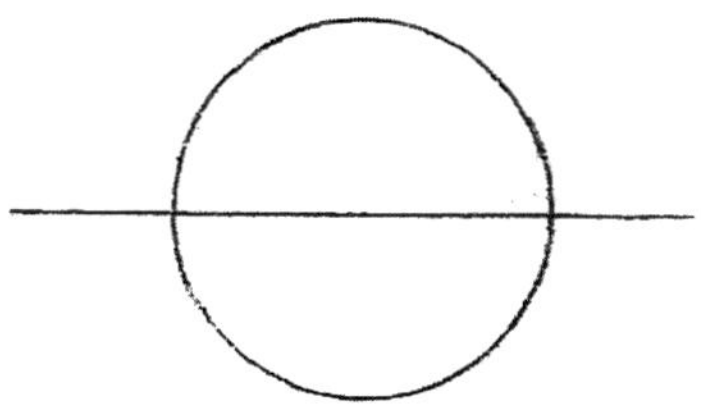

(d)

Up to one turn of 360 degrees in the horizontal plane, for passing and the DEFINING MOMENT OF THE FINAL BALL.

Fig. 6 – 6 (a) (b) (c) and (d)

Passing and Crossing - using the path of least resistance – inter- pass and interchange

Perfect Practice side-foot, slide rule, one touch, silky smooth, fluent on the turf, pass with exquisite timing – look up – to the nearest team-mate: then team-mate to team-mate, pass and move going forward, using the path of least resistance - keep it flowing - DO NOT PASS TO THE OPPONENT during the game.
The side of the foot is the most accurate, and consistent way to make a pass. The outside of the foot is also used to direct the ball to its destination, but requires more skill and Perfect Practice to get it right, and to keep it right.

Strings of UNBROKEN slide rule passes and crosses, right down to the DEFINING MOMENT OF THE FINAL BAL – this is another form of in-play defending.
Before you pass or cross a ball – look up – pass and move quickly with strings of UNBROKEN passes.
Passing and moving quickly does not give the opponent time to close you down or get to the ball first – in this way you are able to keep possession longer. Some players tend to make stray passes or give the ball to the opponent – this must be avoided, if good possession is to be maintained.
Sometimes you may have to ride tackles from the opponent, as you pass and move – be prepared for this situation- always pass and move with a particular GOAL SCORING move in mind.
Do not over-hit the pass or cross and do not under-hit the pass or cross – remember just before the impact with the ball is the foot or the head velocity, and the line of action of the force.
Do not make aimless passes and crosses during training and on match days.
Passing and crossing requires common sense, brain to boot – head co-ordination and ball dynamics which means complete ball control.

A good pass could win you the game: a bad pass could lose you the game.
Passing to an UNMARKED team-mate in splendid isolation is the best passing option.
Use 80% - 90% one touch side-foot slide rule on the turf passes to team-mates, and 10% - 20% long ball.
Long balls are more difficult to control, and often go astray. It can be used as an OVER THE TOP element of surprise through ball for a forward moving team–mate to latch on to and score.

Inter-Passing and Interchanging Configurations - Defence Splitting Shapes

Angular, triangular, passing, moving and dribbling in the horizontal plane - on the turf and some crosses and passes can be done in the vertical plane – these are more difficult to control.

Passing: exchanging passes: inter-passing: interchanging: squaring a pass and implementing the DEFINING MOMENT OF THE FINAL BALL.

One or more "HOLD UP" players to get in the opponent 18 yd box with participating team-mates to implement this special move. The spot in the following figures represents the positions of the team–mates with respect to the various angles, and velocity in which the ball is moved around to confuse the opponents.

PASS AND MOVE

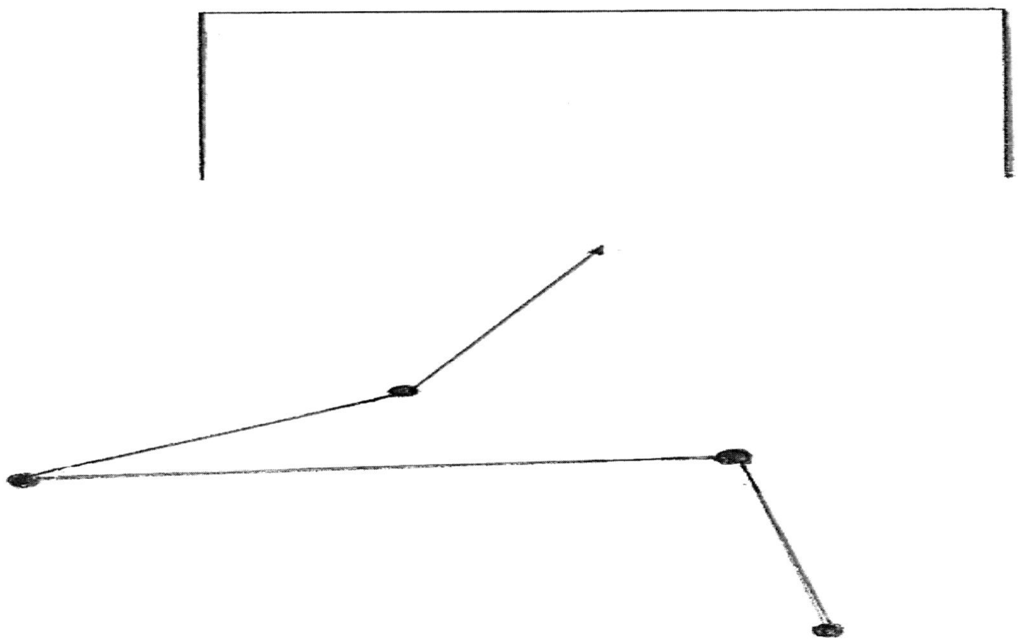

Fig. 7 – 6 (a) angular

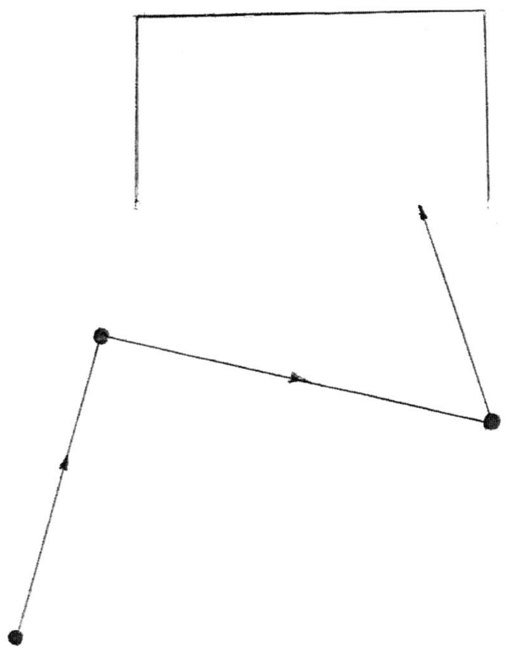

PASS AND MOVE

Fig. 7 – 6 (b) angular

To produce a silky smooth, side-foot, slide rule on the turf, well timed one touch pass, cross or head strike requires the following stages when in possession of the ball.

Pass in the Horizontal Plane

1. Look up for the UNMARKED team-mate in splendid isolation.
2. Look for the COMPLETE SPACE – THE PATH OF LEAST RESISTANCE.
3. CENTRE OF GRAVITY of the player must be within the base for on the turf passes.
4. The player's FOOT VELOCITY to give the ball the correct impact during set-play or in-play.
The player foot angles, that is, side-foot 90 degrees to the ball, is the angle between the radius and tangent of the ball for a 90 degrees pass, and an acute foot angle for less than 90 degrees pass in the horizontal plane – on the turf, Figs. 18 – 6 (a) – shows the line of action of the force - remember the line of action of the force gives you the angle to strike.
5. The ball must reach the team-mate with slide rule accuracy, and with the least amount of difficulty, so that he / she can control it quickly, easily and not lose possession.

90 degrees side-foot, slide rule on the turf is used for normal passing. The outside of the boot is, also at times, used for some element of surprise passes.

Body turn can be used to increase or decrease foot angles by swivelling on the other foot.

Horizontal to Vertical Plane – Surface to Air

For other passes such as longer – higher over the top in the vertical plane – in the air the ANGLE OF ELEVATION which is the acute angle with the turf horizontal. The centre of gravity of the player should be slightly outside the base, to give the ball lift, the height of the lift will depend on the degree to which the centre of gravity is altered or the amount of lean back the player implements before he / she strikes the ball.

From a Cross using a leap and head velocity.

For knock down or knock back headers from a cross in the vertical plane, the ANGLE OF DEPRESSION is used – and this is the acute angle with the eye horizontal projecting downwards – see right and left wingers in Chapter 4, and Fig 22 – 6 (b).

From a Pass or a Cross using a leap and head velocity.

Obtuse headed angle more than 90 degrees, but less than 180 degrees – nearer the 180 degrees for producing a low strike with the head, and nearer the 90 degrees for high strike with the head in the vertical plane- see obtuse angle strike in Fig. 27 – 6 (a) (b).

The shortest distance, to a team-mate is a straight line. If you side-foot a ball, on the turf to a team-mate: this must be done by striking the ball at 90 degrees, with the side of the foot. Assuming other conditions, such as the centre of gravity of the player's body – foot angles – smooth pitch –weather, the foot velocity, and the line of action of the force are right – the ball should travel in a straight line to the team-mate. Balls that are not on the turf, such as rising, falling or coming at various heights and angles, will have to be controlled before the pass is made, use Newton's first law of motion.

The same applies to striking the ball with the head – getting the angles of the head in relation to the ball right, so the ball hits the target. This requires good timing – use of leap velocity, and height of leap - the head velocity and the line of action of the force. Factors such as centre of gravity – velocity – acceleration – impact – momentum, are basically described in Chapter 5, and will help players to gain more confidence in their Perfect Practice.

One touch – unbroken passing – moving and riding tackles QUICKLY – right down to implementing the DEFINING MOMENT OF THE FINAL BALL – reduces the capacity of the opponents to close you down because in this way you do not give them time and complete space.

Side-footing a football with the side of the foot for a footballer, is similar to a golfer, using his putting club to put the ball into the hole, requires slide rule accuracy and line of action of the force.

Head angles, varied, dependent on the heights and angles of crosses:

Possession – Perfect Practice - ten to twenty unbroken passes at a time is a good string.

Possession in football / soccer is to keep the ball – individually or collectively for as long as possible. Possession consists of complete ball control, and accurate passing. Keeping the ball for far longer periods, than the opponents during the 90 minutes, plus extra time is GOOD TIGHT POSSESSION but make it worthwhile by scoring goals.
Strings of UNBROKEN slide rule passes and crosses, right down to DEFINING MOMENT OF THE FINAL BALL using the path of least resistance – pass and move quickly, interchanging, inter-passing and exchanging passes with team-mates, look up before making a slide rule pass or cross to a team-mate. Good understanding and co-ordination between team-mates are essential for this type of interplay.

Possession is, also about energy conservation. If you lose the ball, you have to work that much harder to win it back: which means you have wasted a lot of energy in trying to win the ball back; energy that will be so useful towards the last ten minutes, plus extra time of the game – it also gives the opponent chances to score.

So, do not give the ball to the opponents: do not lose the ball by being careless, and this includes the goalkeeper. Possession is 11 team-mates with the ball at any point in time during the game.

Riding a Tackle

Sometimes the opponents are unable to win games, because your team is playing consistently better – so they revert to rough stuff tactics. The rough stuff tactics may be intentional, or unintentional – and the degree of intent may vary; some may be less serious: others may be more serious which could put a player out for a long period of time. This is a difficult situation, and requires total discipline from the player and team-mates. It also requires that the player possess a high degree of skill to ride the opponent tackle. The player must be able to quickly leap or raise his / her feet away or over the opponent feet, and not get caught or tangled with the opponent: the player must also stay on his / her feet while in control of the ball, so as to keep possession: quick reaction and response, eyes behind your head, so to speak, to help combat this type of rough stuff tackle, Fig 16 – 6.

Riding a Tackle

Fig. 16 – 6: feet movement away from the opponent – but still in control of yourself and the ball, so that you do not lose possession and continue with strings of unbroken passing and moving.

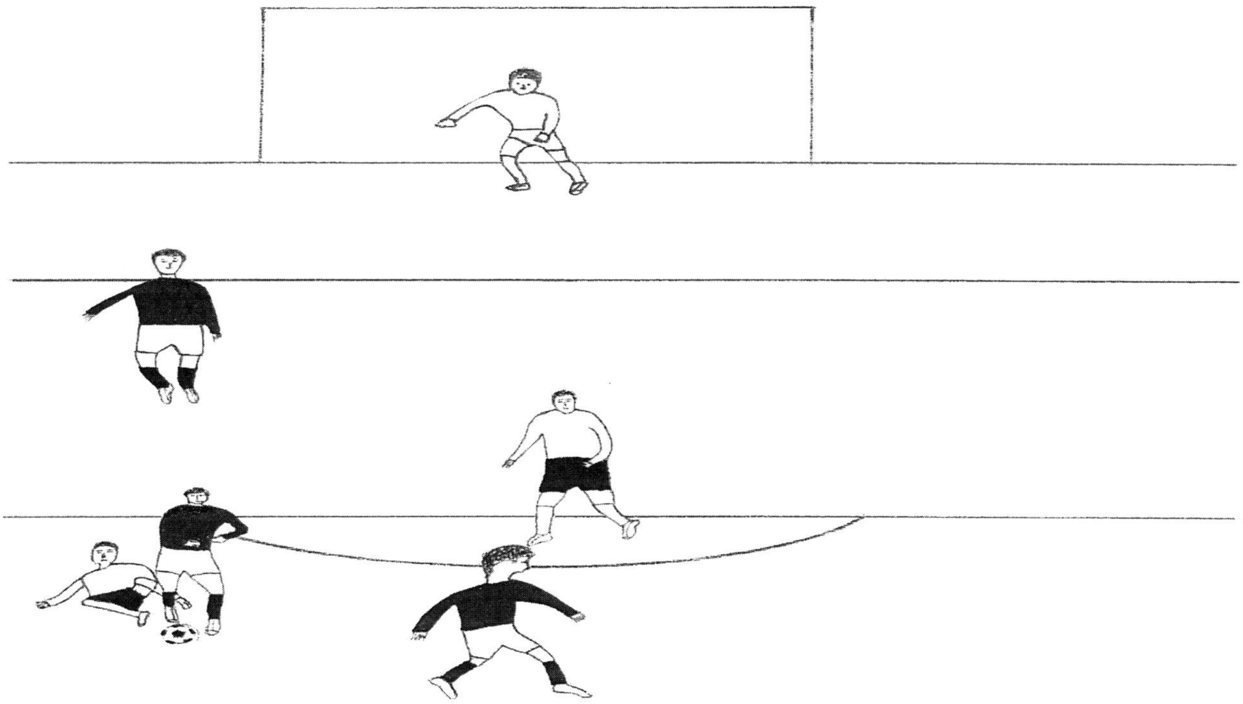

THE PRODUCTION OF-
THE DEFINING MOMENT OF THE OF THE FINAL BALL IN THE HORIZONTAL PLANE - on the turf – AND VERTICAL PLANE – in the air – remember, power is no good without precision. Once the chance is created, the DEFINING MOMENT OF THE FINAL BALL requires TIME and COMPLETE SPACE – CONTROL then STRIKE the ball.

CHANCE is a created opportunity to implement the DEFINING MOMENT OF THE FINAL BALL.

TIME and COMPLETE SPACE – when you have the ball, there are no opponent close to you – this is the path of least resistance – from the moment of contact with the ball, right down to the ball entering the opponent net – no players should be in the way – including the goalkeeper. The final ball is the ultimate pass or cross with the feet or head, and must be of slide rule accuracy.
To help the players create COMPLETE SPACE for the final ball in the opponent 18 yd area, it will be necessary to implement – quicker passing and moving - angled cut back or pull back – angular and triangular inter-passing and interchanging – exchanging passes – turning opposing defenders through various angles in the horizontal plane – over the top cross or pass – direct, and indirect free kicks – knock down or knock back headers – body swerve to dummy opponents – back heel – long throws – chest down and line up ball – juggling with the ball, dummy and chip the goalkeeper: the final obstacle is the opponent goalkeeper, and the final ball must be placed outside his / her reach, that is, the largest SPACE between the goalkeeper, the post, and under the bar. Do not kick the ball straight at the opponent goalkeeper – this is a waste of time and energy. If the goalkeeper moves to quickly to stop the ball, then there is nothing you can do about it.
CONTROL is about the player's centre of gravity, characteristic points, and striking the angles in relation to the ball, and target – and the application of Newton's first law of motion.

STRIKE is the boot or head velocity before impact with the ball – also included in the strike is the LINE OF ACTION OF THE FORCE on the ball – which determines the STRIKE ANGLES, in the horizontal and vertical planes. Fig 5 –6, Fig. 18 – 6 (a) and Fig. 19 – 6 (a) – the anchor/pivot foot helps the player to control his/her centre of gravity, and to give leverage to the kicking foot.

Some players score goals easily, some find it difficult, and some never scores at all. To remove the fear factor, and obtain confidence, consistency, and continuity, players should approach the final ball in the following way.

First the chance to score must be created – this is half of it. The other half is, at the same time to automatically, and instinctively create the TIME and COMPLETE SPACE and CONTROL which consists of the body's centre of gravity, Newton's first law of motion – boot or head striking angles, and velocity – with chosen characteristic point on the boot or head to the chosen characteristic point on the ball, and with the correct impact STRIKE the ball cleanly past the opponent goalkeeper. The striker has only a split second in which to gather these factors together, before he / she strikes the ball. This is the DEFINING MOMENT OF THE FINAL BALL IN the HORIZONTAL and VERTICAL PLANES.
Fig. 1-7 shows where the ball should be placed in the "GO" area, and to avoid the "NO GO" area at all times. If one of these factors is not correct, it will affect the direction, and outcome of the final ball.
Remember –

CHANCE + TIME & COMPLETE SPACE + CONTROL + STRIKE

Created

no opponents near including the goalkeeper

before the impact is the boot, or head velocity and the line of action of the force

Newton's first law of motion, chosen C. G of player – chosen head, or boot angle - chosen characteristic point on the boot, or head to the chosen characteristic point on the ball

If there is no TIME or COMPLETE SPACE or both, then hold on to the ball – move the ball around, inter–change, inter-pass and exchange passes with team-mates, until you could create TIME and COMPLETE SPACE to fully implement the DEFINING MOMENT OF THE FINAL BALL.

Scoring goals against any opponent – especially a strong one is not easy – but it will become easier with plenty of Perfect Practice, using the DEFINING MOMENT OF THE FINAL BALL in both the HORIZONTAL and VERTICAL PLANES.

The ball when struck with the side of the foot is the safest way to score goals in the horizontal plane. Use of other parts of the foot to score goals, such as the toe, inside and outside of the toe are more difficult to control the ball for direction, and slide rule accuracy, because the surface area of the inside, and outside of the toe area is smaller than the side of the foot. The lace area has a good surface area, but control in keeping the ball down must be at its best, that is, the body's centre of gravity must be slightly forward or sideways to get on top of the ball before striking it to keep it down – the lace area is best applied to balls off the turf surface as a safety measure.

The Horizontal and Vertical Planes

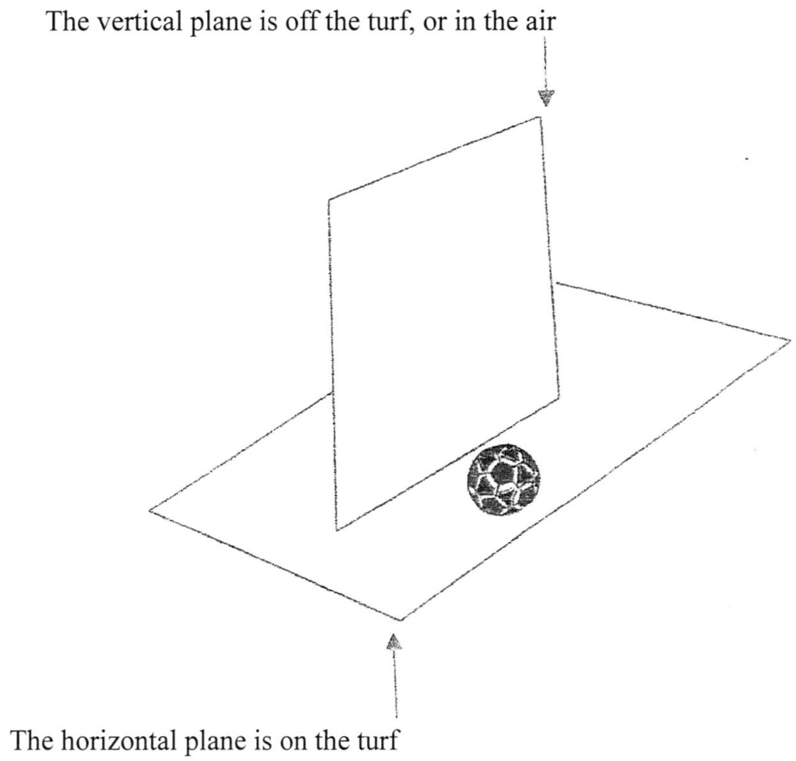

A good team defend, and attack in the horizontal and vertical planes.

Fig. 17 – 6

The Defining Moment Of The Final Ball In The Horizontal Plane – on the turf

(a) **Right angle Strike** – the centre of gravity of the player determines the result of the DEFINING MOMENT OF THE FINAL BALL – the player must be able to adjust to his / her centre of gravity to suit the appropriate foot angle strike in this case a 90 degrees strike to the goal line, and within the limits of the two post and the goalkeeper, Fig. 18 - 6 (a) and 18 – 6 (b).

Side-foot, slide rule on the turf strike – the angle between the radius and tangent is 90 degrees, for passing, taking a penalty and implementing the DEFINING MOMENT OF THE FINAL BALL.

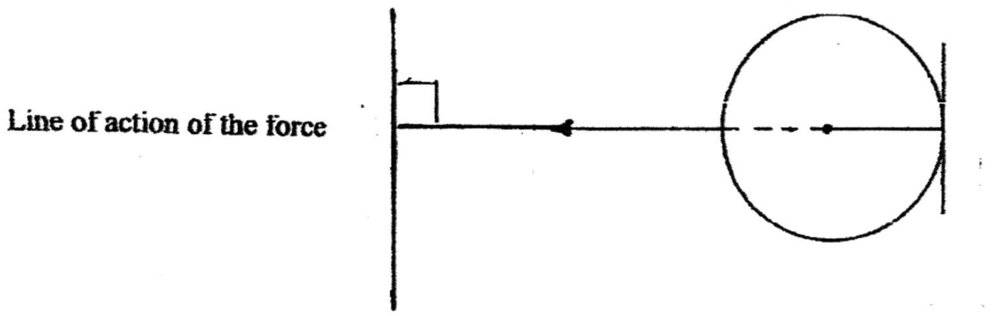

Fig. 18 – 6 (a)

Acute Angle Strike – the centre of gravity of the player must be adjusted as above, and in this case the side-foot, slide rule on the turf strike, is to strike the ball at less than 90 degrees to the goal line, and within the limits of the two posts, and the goalkeeper, Fig. 19 – 6 (a) and Fig. 19 – 6 (b).

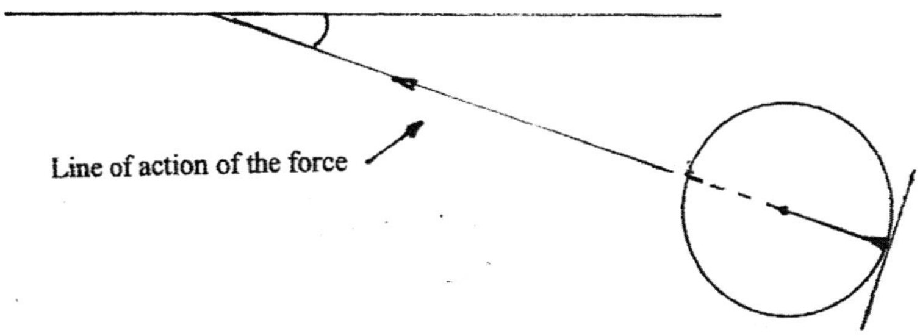

Fig. 19 – 6 (a)

90 Degrees Strike

Fig. 18 – 6 (b): side-foot slide rule on the turf

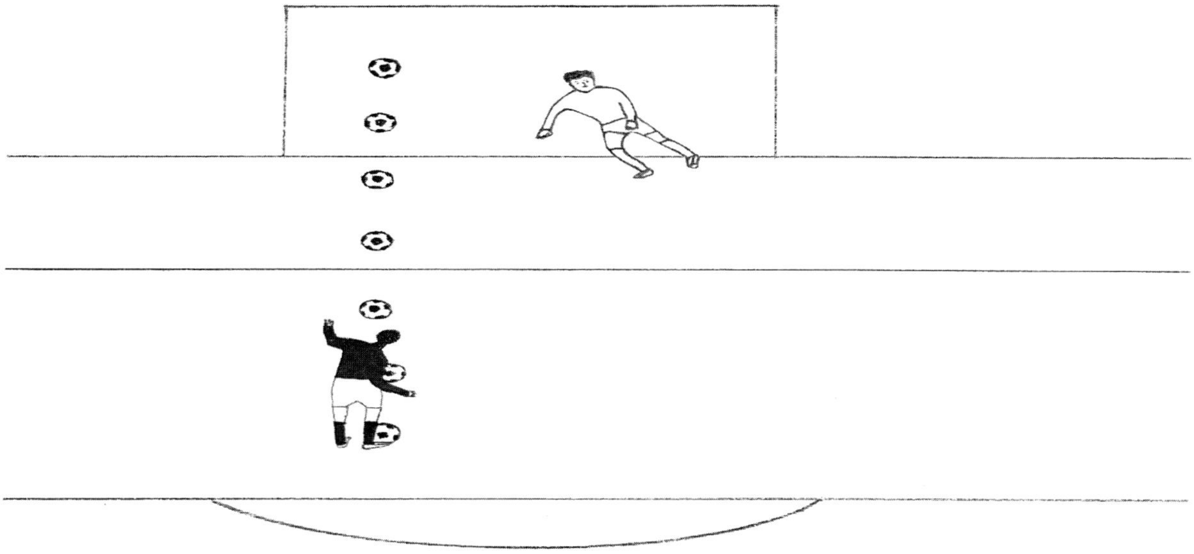

Acute Angle Strike

Fig. 19 – 6 (b): side-foot slide rule on the turf

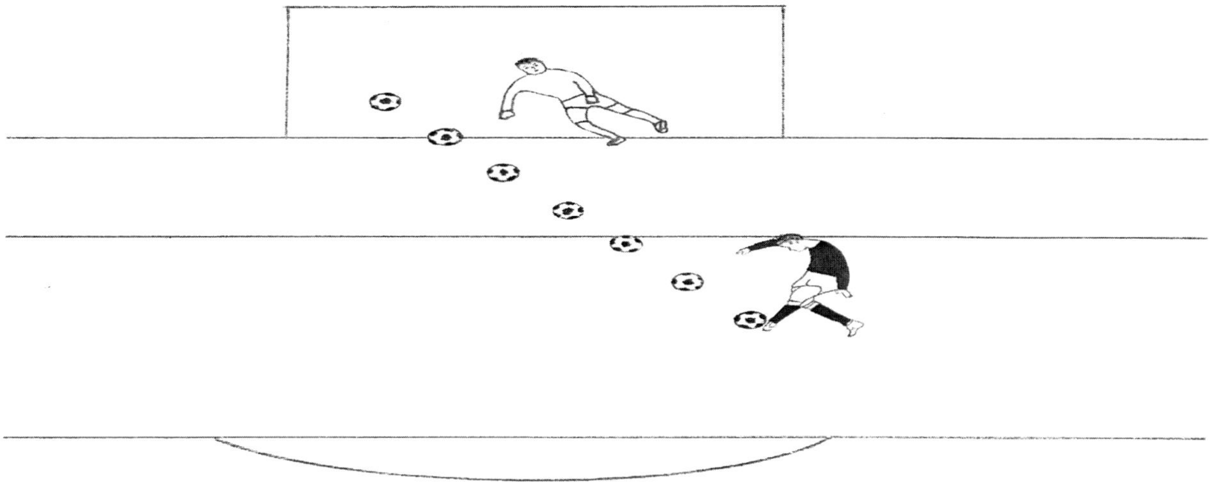

The Angle Of Elevation Strike – ball kicked from on the turf to in the air – that is the horizontal to the vertical plane - Surface to air.

In Fig. 20 – 6 (a) and (b), if the ball is kicked from the angles, and distances shown, the chances are that the ball may rise above the bar – it may hit the bar or it may go under the bar, this set up is tight and risky – also there are other factors to consider such as impact, drag force, air properties, kinetic energy, dip etc,.

In Fig. 20 – 6 (c) and (d), gives a safety factor of approximately 1 ft or 0.91m below the bar to aim for. A theoretical safe strike would be between 5 and 7 degrees for 15 to 25 yd or 13.6 to 19 .1m. 8 degrees for 9 to 15 yd or 8.1 to 13.6 m, and 15 to 25 degrees for 3 to 9 yd or 2.7 to 8.1m In general 7 degrees or less will cover 25 yd or 22.7 m and under safely – the ball cannot go lower than the turf, but it can go higher, if it is not controlled – a good reason to keep the ball nearer the turf.

A trial and error method will have to be employed with Perfect Practice by the players to get the shooting angles and distances right – and this includes the implementation of the DEFINING MOMENT OF THE FINAL BALL for the angle of elevation strike.

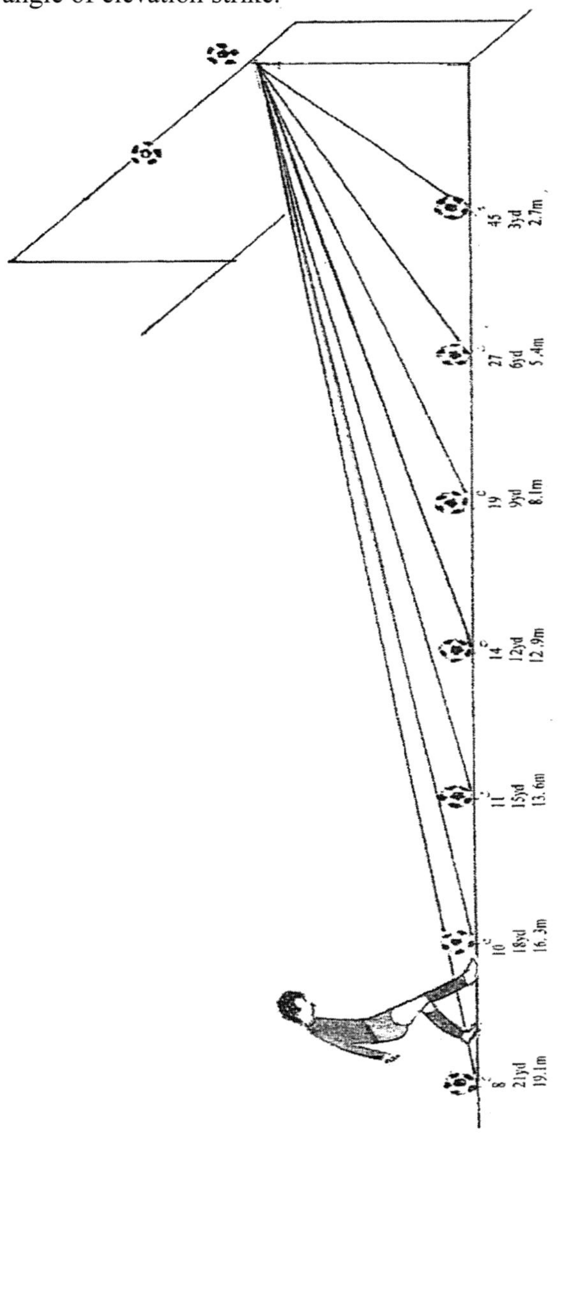

UNRESTRICTED ANGLE OF ELEVATION STRIKE - SURFACE TO AIR

Fig.20 – 6(a)

Unrestricted Angle of Elevation Strike – Surface To Air

Fig. 20 – 6 (b) for a strike that needs to give the ball more lift – the C.G. of the player has to be altered to give more lean back same as Fig. 20 – 6 (a) – with respect to angles and distances.

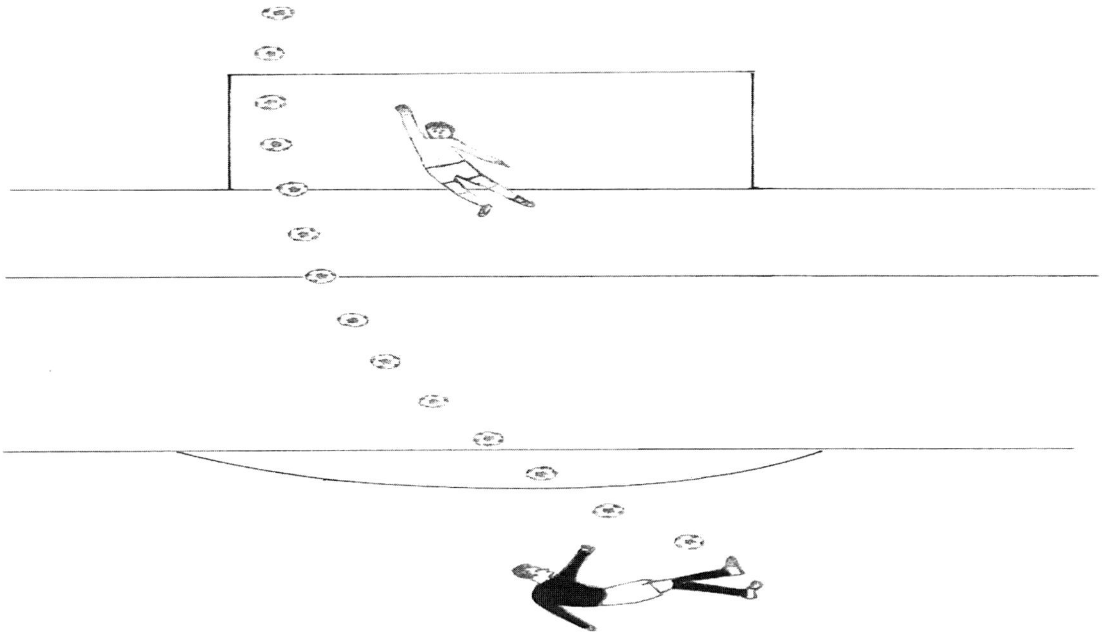

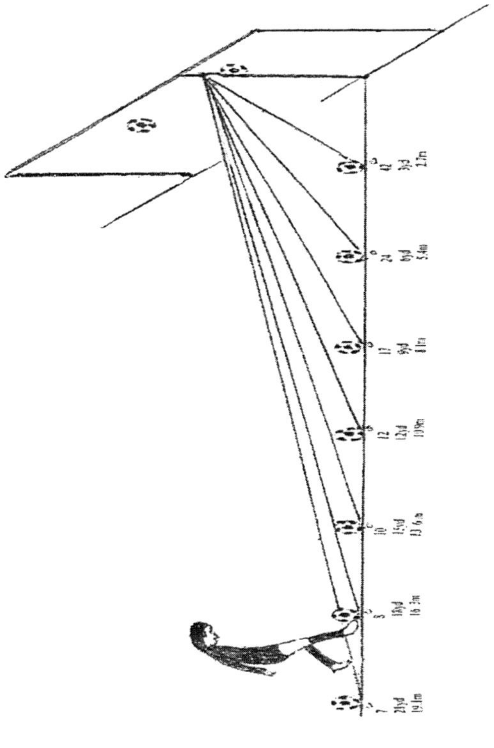

RESTRICTED ANGLE OF ELEVATION STRIKE-SURFACE TO AIR

Fig.20 -6(c)

Restricted Angle of Elevation Strike – Surface to Air

Fig. 20 – 6 (d) for a strike that needs a small lift and small alteration of player's C.G. same as Fig. 20 – 6 (c) – with respect to angles and distances.

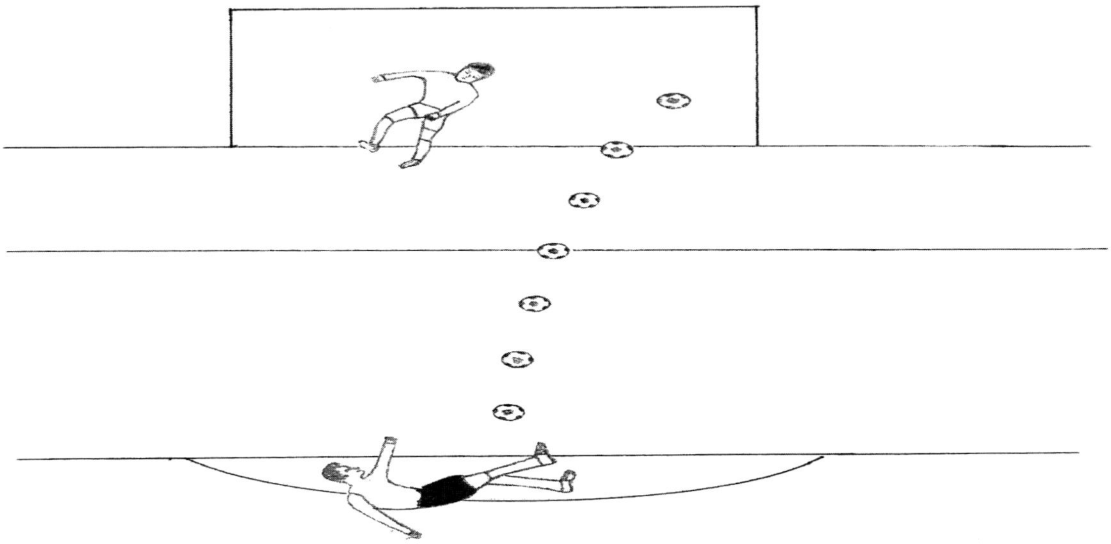

The Defining Moment of the Final Ball in the Horizontal to Vertical Plane – Surface to Air

Foot Strike – Restricted Angles of Elevation and Distance – Fig. 20 – 6 (a) (b)

Foot Strike – Restricted Angles of Elevation and Distances

Angle Of Elevation – to strike the ball at an angle with the turf horizontal – safe strike angles varies between 0 and 7 degrees for distances from 5 metres to 25 metres.
The angle of elevation in this instance is to keep the ball within the limits of the two goal posts – beneath the bar – the turf – and outside the reach of the goalkeeper. Fig 20 – 6 (c) (d)

Remember the PRODUCTION of the DEFINING MOMENT OF THE FINAL BALL.

When the player is satisfied that he / she has all the factors under control, the player has only a split second in which to do so – then the player can strike the ball into the net.

The Horizontal and Vertical Planes

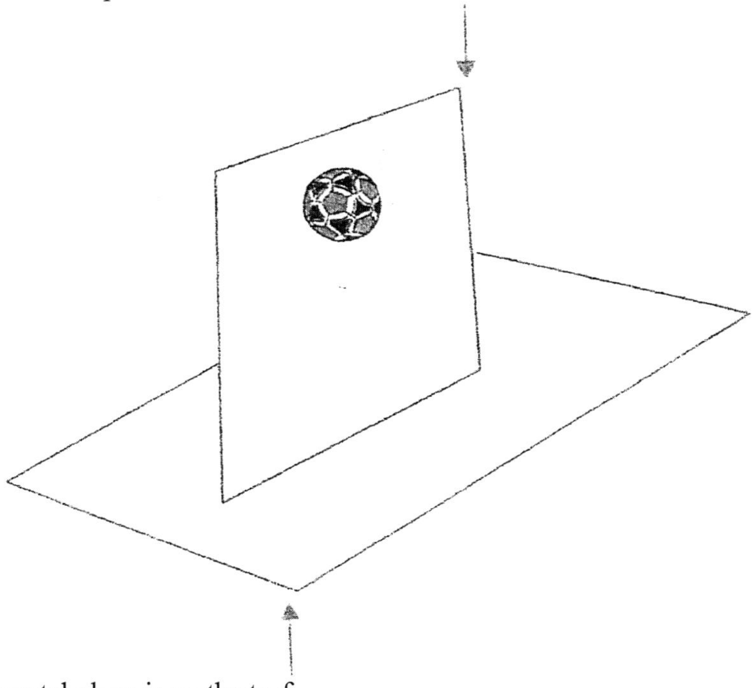

Fig. 21 - 6

Head Angles Strike of the Ball in the Vertical Plane – ball in the air.

Safety Note – players must know his / her heading limitations before attempting to head high velocity crosses – see impact in Chapter 5.

(a) Acute Angle of Depression
(b) Obtuse Restricted Angle
(c) Acute - restricted Head or Boot Angle

(a) Acute Angle of Depression for leaping, knock down or knock back headers, Fig. 22 – 6(a)

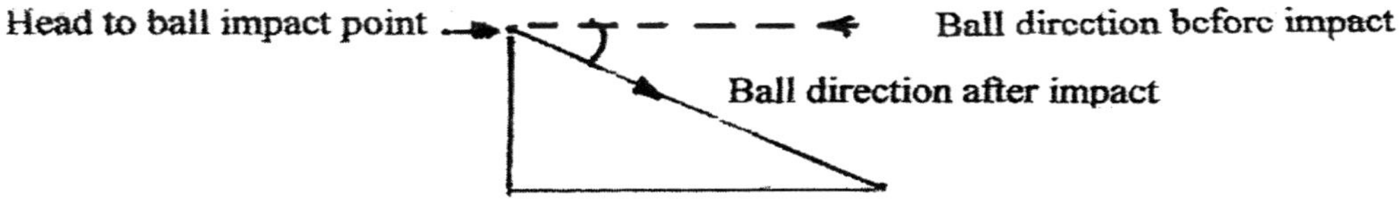

Knock Down or Knock Back Headers are based on Aim and Impact – line of action of the force.

The acute angle of depression is the angle between the eye sight horizontal and the line of direction of the ball after impact with the player's head as it enters the opponent net – knocked down to an UNMARKED team–mate, knocked down for a goal mouth scramble: or knocked back to an UNMARKED team-mate in splendid isolation: in the opponent 18 yd / penalty area.
Good timing in leaping for the ball – the leap velocity and height are essential for the player to get his head and body's centre of gravity at the correct angle: to get on top of the ball to keep it down: again controlling these angles, will help the strikers to direct the ball, to within the limits of the two goal posts - under the bar

and the goalkeeper. Before the impact is the head velocity – at impact is the line of action of the force: gives direction. Some header's requires the player's centre of gravity and head angle to be altered; for example a diving header where the player has to move forward to make contact with the ball to keep it down, and direct it into the opponent net.

When a team-mate makes a downward header strike into the opponent penalty area for a scramble, the impact and angle of the head onto the ball must be such that the ball strikes the turf at the correct distance from the goal line: so that the ball does not bounce over the bar – keeping in mind the hardness or softness of the turf – if the ball does bounce over the bar the striker's impact and angle with the turf is wrong – if the ball is knocked down directly into the opponent net and hits the turf past the goal line – as the ball bounces off the turf it will be collected by the net and the opponent goalkeeper, impact angle is right.

Acute Angle Knock Down Header

Fig. 22 – 6(b) from a corner kick acute angle knock down header into the opponent net.

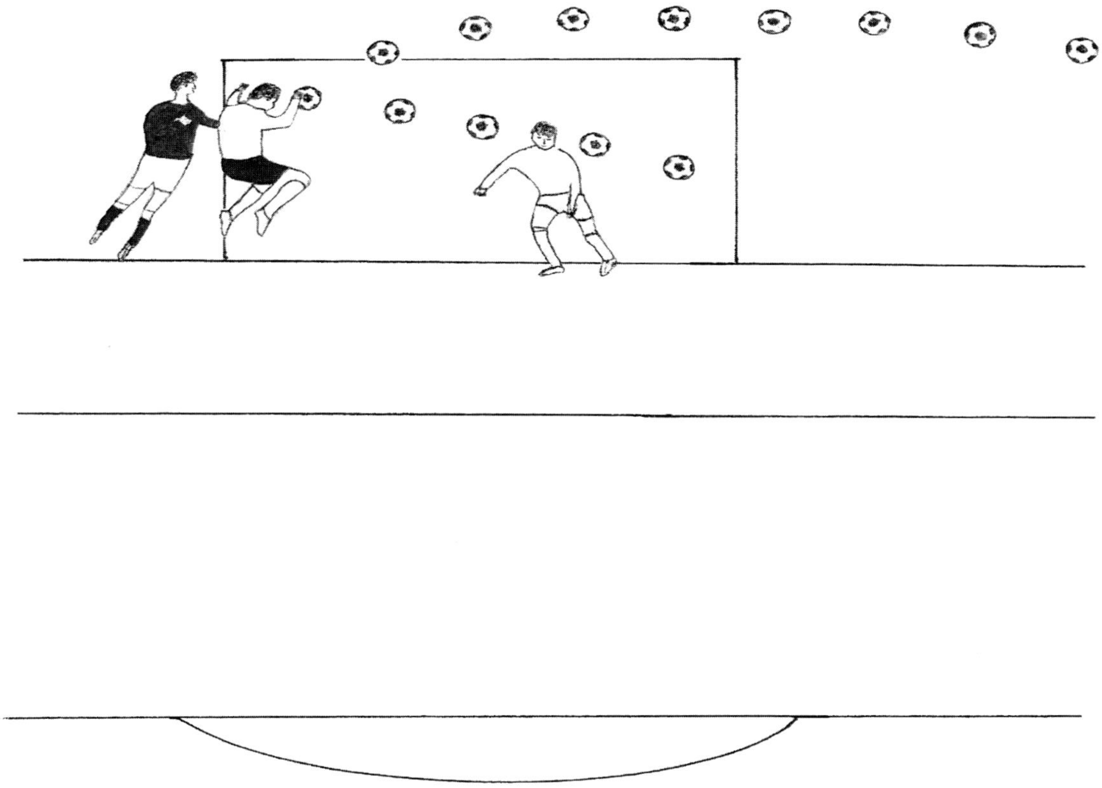

The Corridors of Uncertainty – Tight Angle Areas in the Horizontal and Vertical Planes

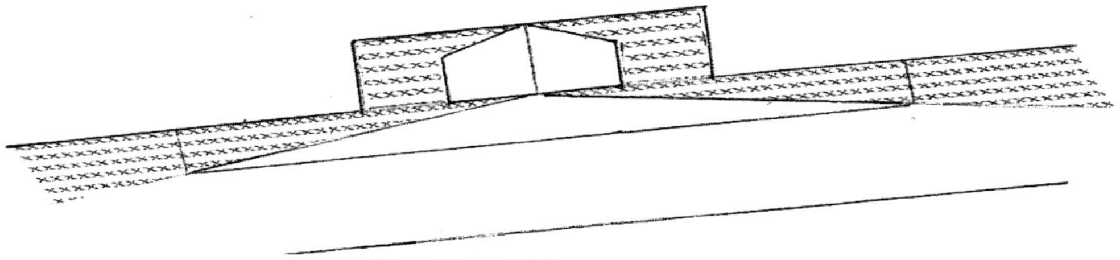

Fig. 23 – 6 (a)

Some opposing defenders will force you into the tight angle area – especially the tightest of angles.
The shaded areas shown in Fig. 23 – 6 (a) is known as the corridors of uncertainty or tight angle area in the horizontal and vertical planes. The angle makes it difficult to obtain complete space due to the opposing goalkeeper and defenders in place.
A strike should only be made if there is COMPLETE SPACE to put the ball into the opponent net, otherwise use a cut back or pull back in the horizontal plane or a knock back header in the vertical plane - or hold on to the ball till complete space is created.

Knock Down or Knock Back Headers – Tight Angles Areas or Corridor in the Vertical Plane

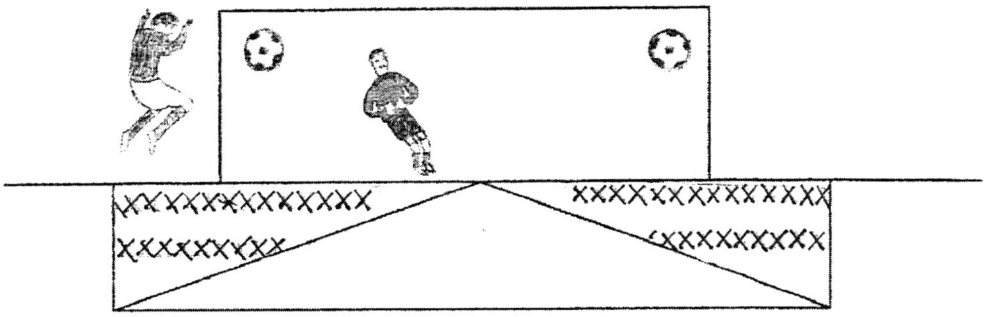

Fig. 23 – 6 (b)

In the vertical plane the striker has a better chance to implement the DEFINING MOMENT OF THE FINAL BALL in the tight angle area or corridor due to more available space – because the goalkeeper cannot spread himself / herself in the vertical plane as he / she can on the horizontal plane.

Theoretical Calculations

Theoretical calculations practices will help the player to gain a better understanding, and mental picture of varied angled knock down, and knock back headers for a scramble or to an UNMARKED team-mate in the opponent18 yd / penalty area.
The trigonometric ratios of sine, cosine and tangent for a right-angled triangle are given as:

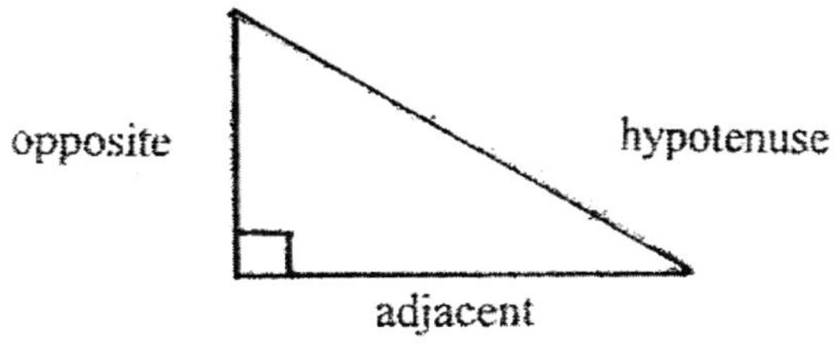

Fig.24 – 6

$$\text{sine } \theta = \frac{\text{opposite}}{\text{hypotenuse}}$$

$$\text{cosine } \theta = \frac{\text{adjacent}}{\text{hypotenuse}}$$

$$\text{tangent } \theta = \frac{\text{opposite}}{\text{adjacent}}$$

If you know one side, and one angle, the other sides can be calculated – and to work out, knock down or knock back distances in the opponent18 yd / penalty area: $\tan\theta = \frac{\text{opposite}}{\text{adjacent}}$

Examples of knock down or knock back distances in the opponent 18 yd / penalty area, using different angles of depression of 45 degrees and 30 degrees are calculated using the right–angled triangle.

$$\tan\theta = \frac{\text{opposite}}{\text{adjacent}}$$

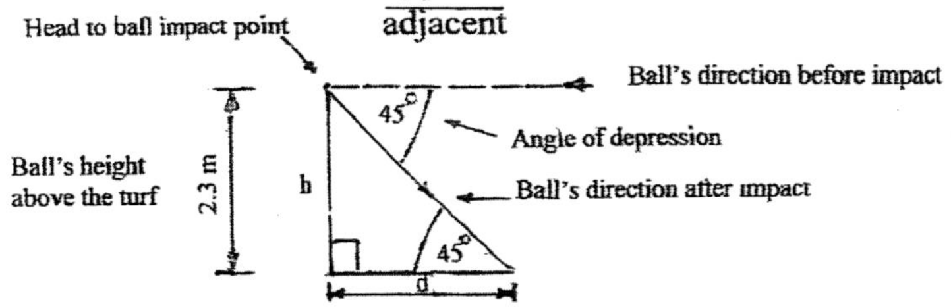

Fig. 25 – 6

We know the height of the ball, as the striker rises to meet it with his head is equal to approximately 2.3 metres. Assuming the striker decides to knock down or knock back the ball using an approximate angle of depression of 45 degrees – this angle is also equal to the alternate angle in the right angled triangle.

From the trigonometric ratio of

$$\tan 45^{\circ} = \frac{2.3}{d}$$

$$\text{then } d = \frac{2.3}{\tan 45^{\circ}}$$

Since from tables or calculator tan 45 degrees is equal to 1

$$\text{Therefore } \frac{2.3}{1} = 2.3 \text{ m.}$$

The ball should drop approximately 2.3 metres in front or at the side of the striker.

If the striker decides to knock the ball directly into the net, knock down for a scramble or knock back to another team-mate at an angle of depression of approximately 30 degrees – this is calculated in the same way as for a 45 degrees strike.

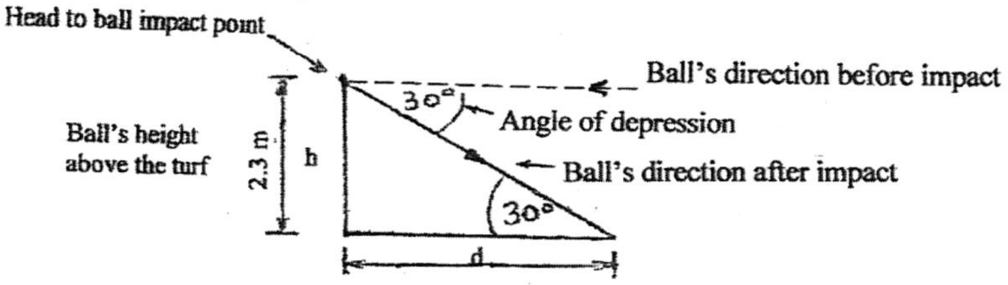

Fig. 26 – 6

Applying $\tan 30^{o} = \frac{2.3}{d}$

Since tan 30 degrees from tables or calculator is equal to 0.5774

$$d = \frac{2.3}{\tan 30^{o}}$$

$$d = 3.98\ m$$

The ball should hit the ground at approximately 4 metres in front or at the side of the striker.

Control of the angles of depression – the striker will be able to pin point his / her headers more accurately, that is, over-hitting or under-hitting headers could be significantly reduced.

The striker will not be able to get angles exact and approximate values will have to be aimed at – but a fair amount of accuracy, will be obtained from trial and error – and Perfect Practice – on the training ground.

The safe knock down angles will depend on – the velocity – the height and direction of the cross – if the player is marked or unmarked – whether the player can get on top of the ball or not – and the correct flick of the head: the player's head velocity.

Striking the ball in the appropriate segment and using the flick of the head will increase or decrease the knock down angles.
For example, if a striker is 1.8 m tall, and rises another 0.3 m to meet the cross, this would give a height of 2.1 m. If the striker gets on top of the ball, and knocks it down – back or directly into the net at approximately 45 degrees downward acute to the eye horizontal, the ball should hit the ground approximately 2 m from the striker – from two equal sides right angle triangle.
By increasing or decreasing the head velocity, angle and body's centre of gravity, in relation to the leap velocity and height of leap the striker will be able to pick the spot to head the ball on with slide rule accuracy.

(b) Obtuse Restricted Head Angle for subtle leaping and Chipping the opponent goalkeeper – when the goalkeeper is off his / her line.

Foot to Head Obtuse Angle Chip and
Foot to Foot Obtuse Angle Chip

Fig. 27 – 6 (a) and Fig. 27 – 6 (b)

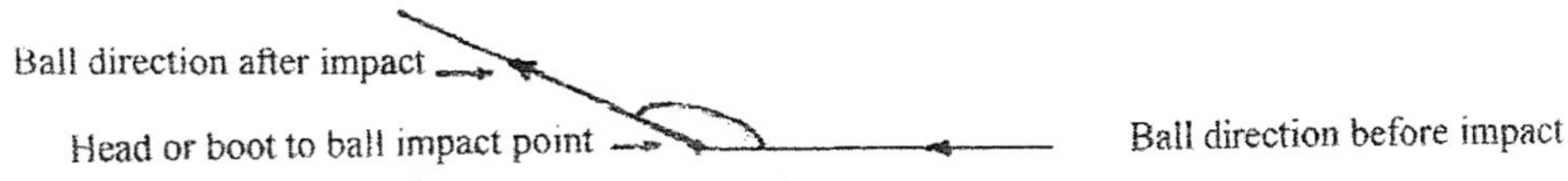

Fig. 27 – 6 (a)

This angle is greater than 90 degrees and less than 180 degrees, and to chip the ball into the opponent net with the subtle use of the head, and the correct impact from the well timed leap requires that the striker to use the angles nearer the 180 degrees slant – this reduces the curvature of the path of the ball; flattens it out so to speak; so that the ball enters the opponent net accurately – that is, within the limits of the two goal posts, under the bar, and the goalkeeper.

Foot to Head Obtuse Angle Chip

Fig. 27 –6 (b) - chip angle nearer the 180 degrees.

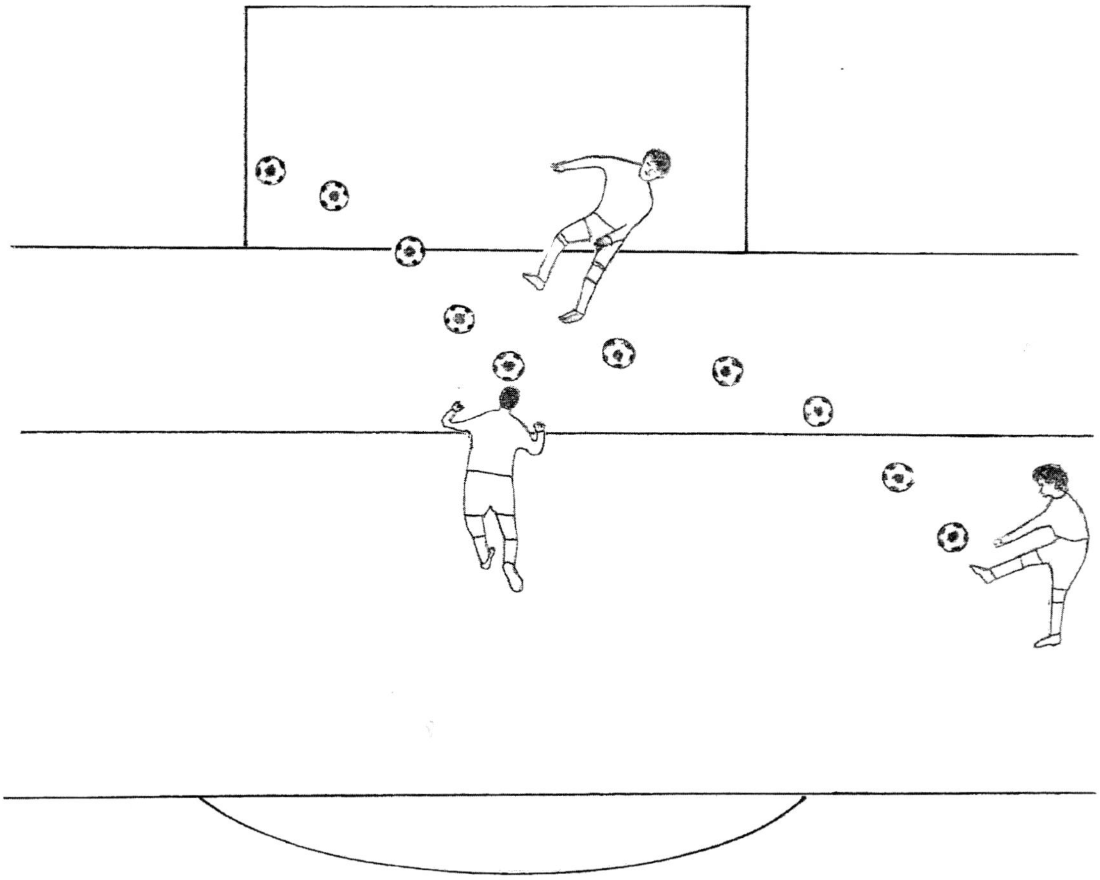

180 degree Chip over Keepers Head

Fig. 28 – 6 and 31 – 6

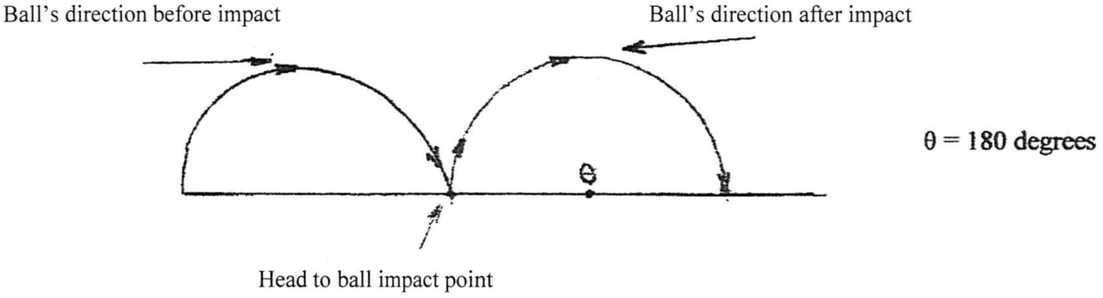

The final ball from a parabolic cross – the ball lands on the top of a team-mate's head who is in or around the opponent 18 yd / penalty area: the team-mate with precise timing and leap gives the ball the correct impact, so that the ball rises and takes the path of a semicircle or goes through 180 degrees over the top of the keeper and in to the net. A striker uses this type of final ball when he / she see the opponent keeper is off his /her line and cannot get back in time.

The foot can also be used to restrict the chip angle and impact of the ball over the keeper's head by implementing the DEFINING MOMENT OF THE FINAL BALL in the vertical plane – in the air.
Fig. 29 – 6 shows foot to foot restricted obtuse angle chip.
Fig. 30 – 6 (b) shows foot to head restricted acute angle chip.
Fig. 31 – 6 shows foot to head to head restricted acute angle chip which can also be converted into a parabolic or semi – circle trajectory over the keeper's head.

Foot to Foot - Restricted Obtuse Angle Chip

Fig. 29 - 6

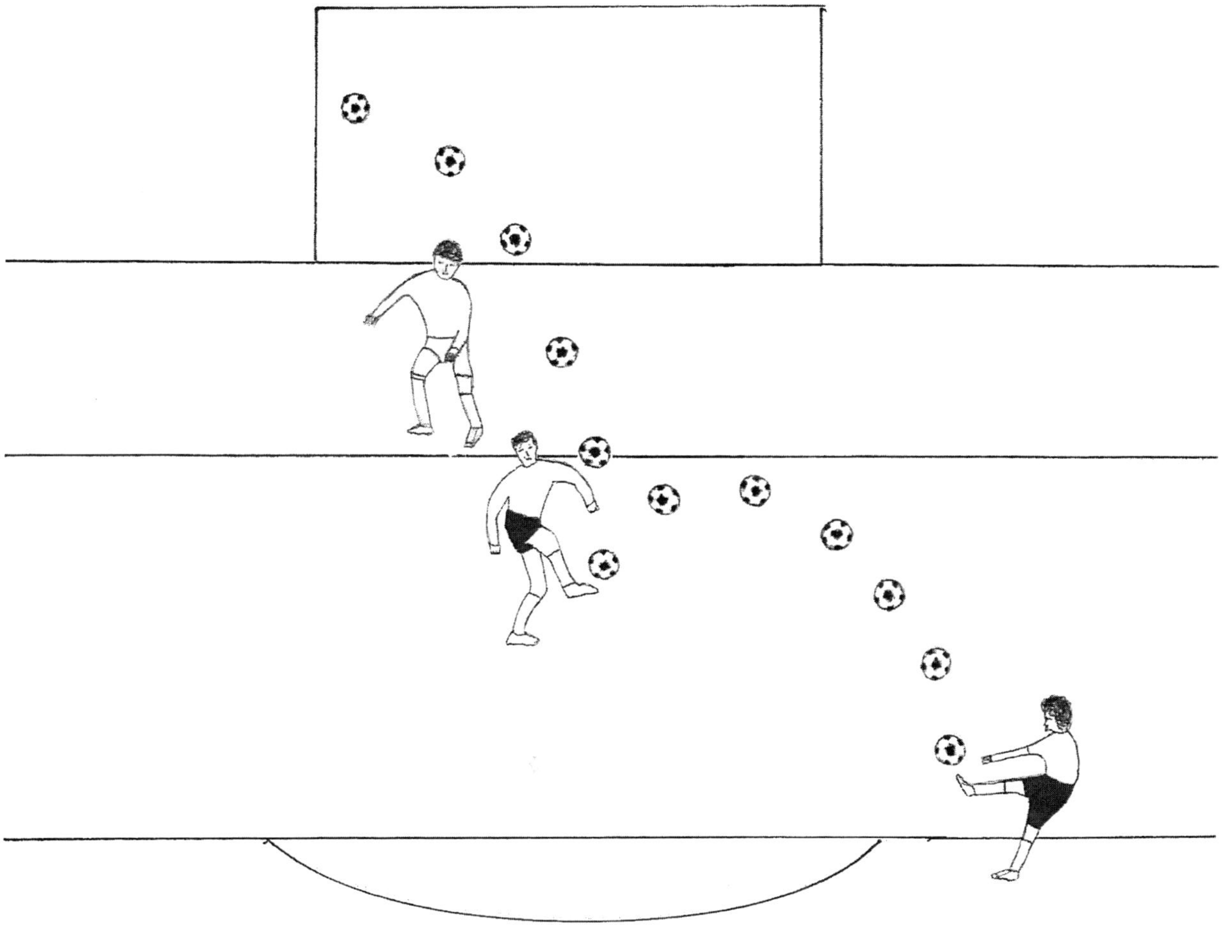

(c) Restricted Acute Head and Foot Angle

Foot to head chip, less than 90 degrees, Fig. 30 – 6 (a) and Fig. 30 – 6 (b).

Foot to head to head chip acute less than 90 degrees, but can also be converted to a 180 degrees parabolic or semi-circle chip over the keeper's head – Fig. 28 – 6 and Fig. 31 – 6.

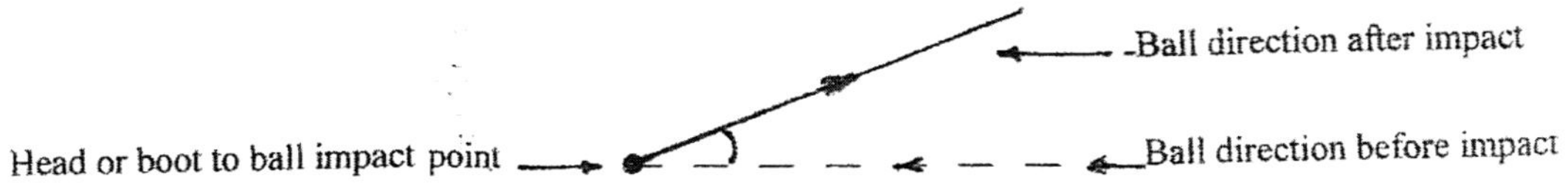

Fig. 30 – 6 (a)

Foot to Head Restricted Acute Angle Chip

Fig. 30 – 6 (b)

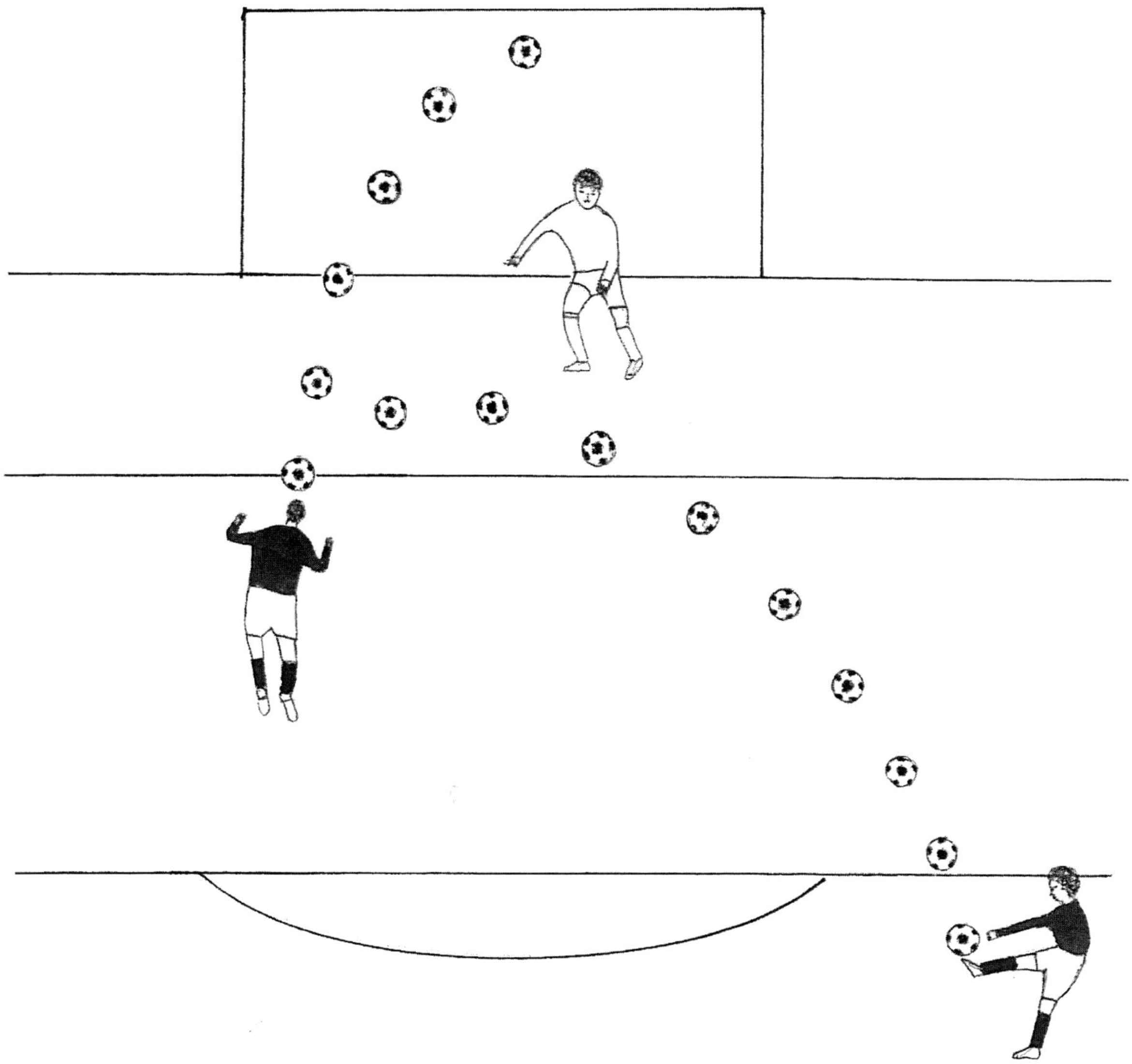

Foot to Head to Head Restricted Acute Angle Chip

Fig. 31 – 6

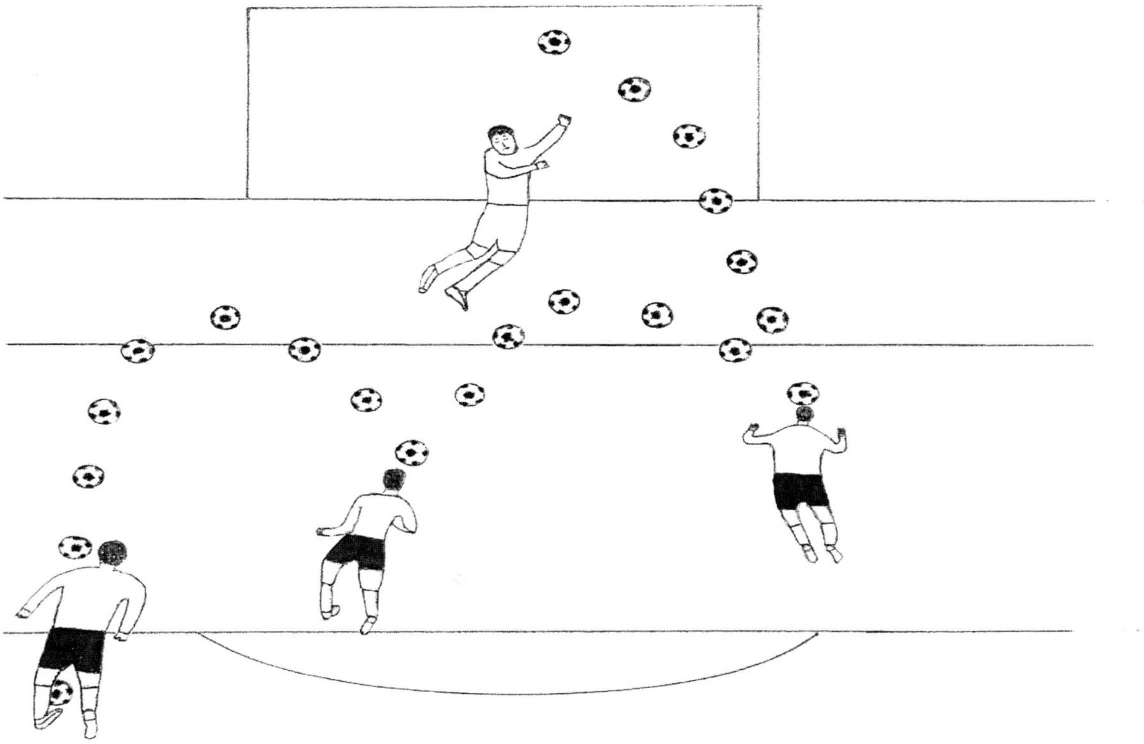

Direct Free Kick

Fig. 32 – 6 a bad wall set up by the opponent – keeper is off his / her line and not in centre of goal – the goalkeeper is selling himself / herself short of time and space – wall is more than 10 m from the ball – the wall is giving too much space to the kicker – so the kicker has a good chance to score.

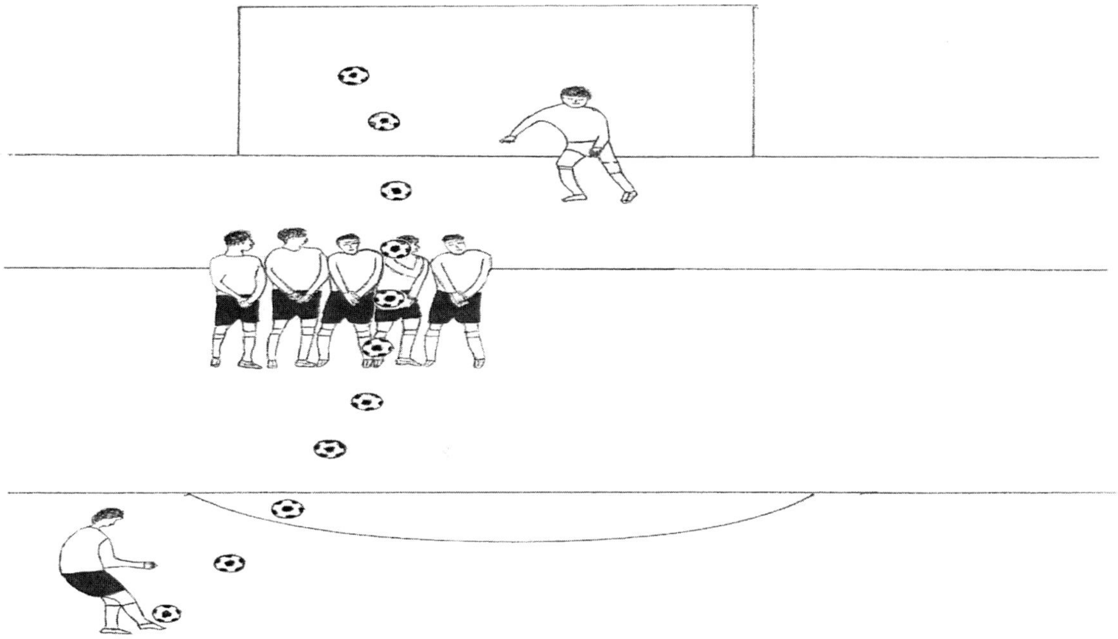

The final ball takes many forms and goes through various conditions – some of which are – from crosses and passes across the face of the opponent goal provided by the wingers. Various headers, 25m long-range drive, interchanging, inter-passing and exchanging passes in the opponent 18 yard / penalty area. Cut back angled passes and crosses from the wingers. Chest down ball - line up and volley in and around the opponent box. Turning defenders –"one and one" with the opponent keeper – sending the opponent keeper the wrong way – chip the opponent keeper - tap in etc,.

The Final Ball under Normal Pressure

The striker should be able to implement the DEFINING MOMENT OF THE FINAL BALL in the horizontal or vertical plane quite easily. The striker's reaction and response should be normal.

The Final Ball under High Pressure

The striker under high pressure is when he or she is being closed down by opposing defenders from all directions and wants to implement the DEFINING MOMENT OF THE FINAL BALL, in this instance the striker must think, and move quickly, that is, his or her reaction and response must be quicker.

Do not panic in the Final Ball Scenario.

Chapter 7

DEFENCE

Closing up Channels

Every player in the team, to Perfect Practice each and everything there is to know, about defending: and how to keep a CLEAN SHEET consistently, with continuity. Remember one point is better than no point.
Remember – if, the opponent cannot score, the opponent cannot win. A CLEAN SHEET = at least 1 point.
Do not INVITE the opponent into your 18yd / penalty area if possible.
The defence is the MOST IMPORTANT department of play, and must be approached, with organisation and discipline - BE TENACIOUS IN DEFENCE - HOLDING BACK 2 must keep their positions.

There are two ways the opponent will attack your defence:

1. DIRECT
2. INDIRECT

1.Direct
- (a) Through the middle.
- (b) Around the sides, and behind the back 3/ 4
- (c) Over the top, including long throws.
- (d) Through a bad wall from a direct free kick.

2.Indirect – lateral thinking.
- (a) Various angled cut back or pull back.
- (b) Overhead kick.
- (c) Back heel.
- (d) Indirect free kick, deflection, disguised pass and a long throw.

The most important factor in DEFENCE is to close down and block off the opponent implementing the DEFINING MOMENT OF THE FINAL BALL in the horizontal and vertical planes by implementing the DEFINING MOMENT IN DEFENCE – in both planes.

Defence - X "NO - GO" Area

Fig. 1 – 7 when implementing the DEFINING MOMENT IN DEFENCE – the ball in not allowed in the X "NO–GO" area – the ball may go to the goalkeeper, over the bar or around the posts.

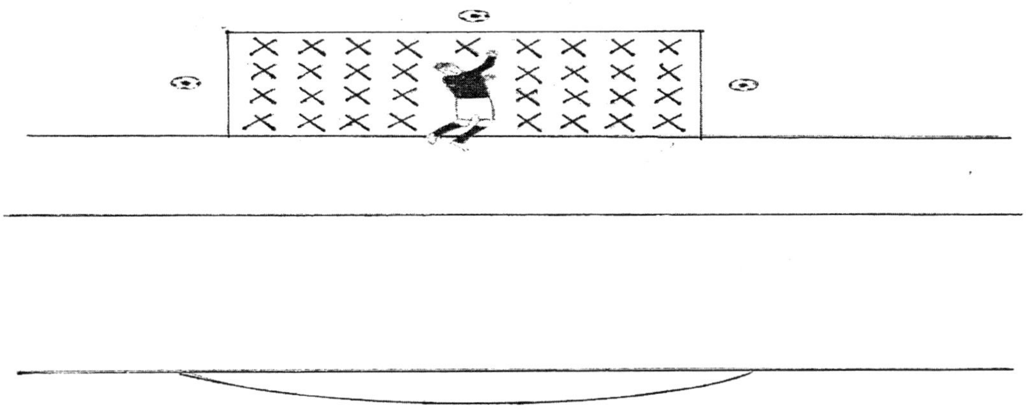

GETTING IN FRONT OF THE OPPONENT DOES NOT MEAN THAT THE OPPONENT IS TOO FAR BEHIND SO AS TO BECOME UNMARKED – IT MEANS CLOSE IN FRONT AND FIRST IN CONTROL OF THE BALL - IN THE HORIZONTAL AND VERTICAL PLANES

Specialist Task for Some Team Players in Defence

Some examples in defence – like defending a set piece corner kick by using your tallest, and best defenders to get in FRONT of the opponents to block them or get to the ball first, to make a safe head clearance: goalkeeper who directs team-mates, and player who are watchful – who watches out for a sneaky UNMARKED opponent in your 18 yd / penalty area and mark them tightly – so that they do not get a free header.

If players are equally good at different tasks – this is even better for the team – this gives the team more options and accuracy – and makes it more difficult for the opponent to cope with.

These SPECIALIST tasks for some players must be statutory, and have Perfect Practice.

A Thin Line between Defence and Attack

When players attack and move forward – although they are attacking – they are also defending – defending the ball while attacking and moving forward, every ball control, passing, possession, right down to the final ball are defended, so the ball ends up in the opponent net, it has to be defended to the end.
When you defend – you defend to the hilt: when you attack you also defend to the hilt – protecting the ball, shielding it from the opponents – keeping it – KEEPING TIGHT POSSESSION.

Defending With a Set of New Players – or Even Well Settled Defenders

Follow the DEFINING MOMENT IN DEFENCE – keep a clean sheet, score a goal, when you get a little better: keep a clean sheet score two goals – that is how to keep a CLEAN SHEET and win.
As your confidence – consistency and continuity gets better then you can turn on the style, and play beautiful football. Do not try to play beautiful football with a poor defence – it will not work well: always make sure your defence standard, and standard of preparation in training, and playing are at their highest peaks.

The Defining Moment In Defence In The Horizontal Plane - on the turf - Statutory

To defend to the end of the game – that is 90 minutes plus extra time requires:

(1) Good understanding amongst team-mates and the goalkeeper.

(2) A PROMPTER - to deal with a potential threat in defence.

Close down the opponent with the ball and close down the UNMARKED opponents at the same time.
The prompter is derived from the “QUEEN HORNET – QUEEN BEE” analogy, is used to PROMPT your reaction and response to defend your 18 yd / penalty area and to keep a clean sheet – to keep you prepared and ready to defend for 90 minutes plus extra time – within the LAWS of the game.
When the queen hornet and queen bee in the hives are threatened, the defending hornets and bees, automatically, and instinctively close in on the opponents, to tackle and block them off and to protect the queen hornet and queen bee from attack. They do this to the hilt, and so defending team-mates must follow this instinctive way of defending to protect their 18 yd / penalty area from the opponents.
Like armed guards ready to repel the opponents from your 18 yd / penalty area, you are prompted by the queen hornet – queen bee analogy to do the same by remembering what they do – back 3/4 and other defenders to give TOTAL PROTECTION to their goalkeeper and the 18yd box.

When an opponent has the ball, it is vital that two or three defending team-mates surround and tackle this opponent, without getting into each other's way to fairly take the ball away from the opponent with a well timed tackle, to block off the opponent, or use safe no hesitation foot clearance, to get rid of the ball out of dangerous area or start a move: go for the ball and not the opponent - do not stand and ball watch - this applies to defending on the turf and in the air. The queen hornet – queen bee analogy consists of prompting your reaction and response – watchful eye, awareness, velocity and acceleration, anticipation, dispossession, tight marking, get in front of the UNMARKED opponent, especially in the 18yd box - get to the ball first, decisive clearances without hesitation or to win possession to start a move – defenders backing up the goalkeeper, with good solid defending, and the goalkeeper watching his/her line backing up the defenders with good solid goalkeeping prompted by the "QUEEN HORNET – QUEEN BEE" analogy, and this is the production of the DEFINING MOMENT IN DEFENCE in the horizontal plane Fig. 2 – 7, in-play.

To stop the opponent from scoring, IN-PLAY defending, in addition this is done as follows:

Deny the opponent TIME and SPACE with early, quick closing down: hassle them, do not let them get to the ball first or settle into any rhythm or game plan – block off the opponents early in midfield, GET IN FRONT OF THE OPPONENTS - to stop any long-range shots.

Mark the opponents – intercept passes, and use careful no hesitation head or feet clearances: use safety first.

Quick, sharp, early closing down is preferably done in the opponent half, so they do not have time and space to build a move in midfield and to stop the opponent from going over the top to score.

In defending, when a player or players run with an opponent who has the ball: running with the opponent is half of it: the other half is to dispossess the opponent fairly, firmly and safely by going for the ball and not the player – with exquisite timing: timing is the key when tackling an opponent.
Do not run with an opponent who has the ball and do nothing – that is a shadow run – a shadow run is a waste of time and energy. Always try to win the ball fairly and make the journey worthwhile.
Win the ball, stay on your feet – keep tight possession.

The Defining Moment in Defence in the Horizontal Plane – on the turf Fig. 2 – 7 when an opponent has the ball – two or three team-mates surround him / her to fairly take the ball away: go for the ball not the opponent, in-play.

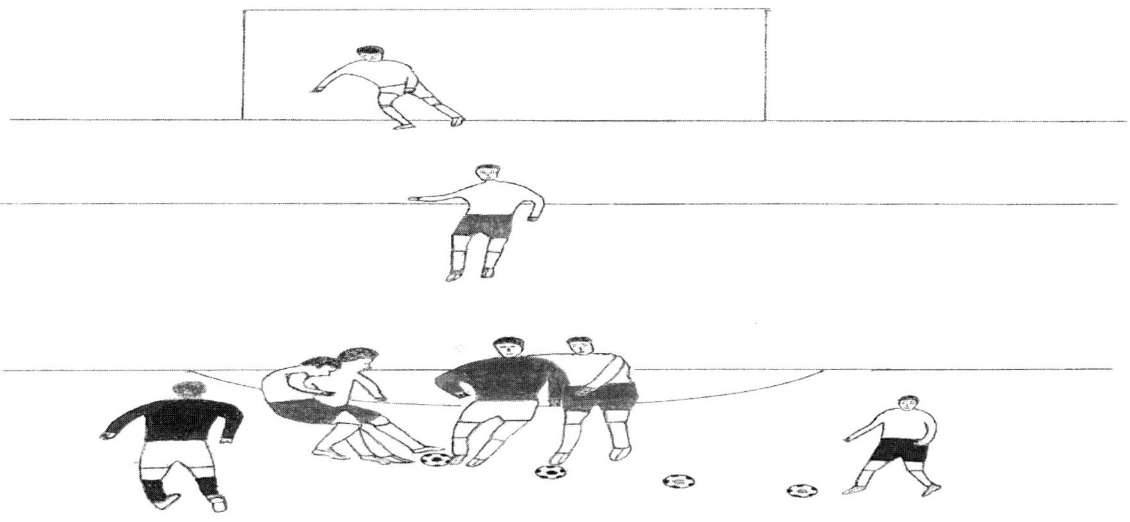

Foot Clearance in the Horizontal Plane – on the turf Fig. 3 – 7 get in front of the opponent for a ball coming across the face of goal and clear safely for a corner or to another part of the pitch or start a move, in-play.

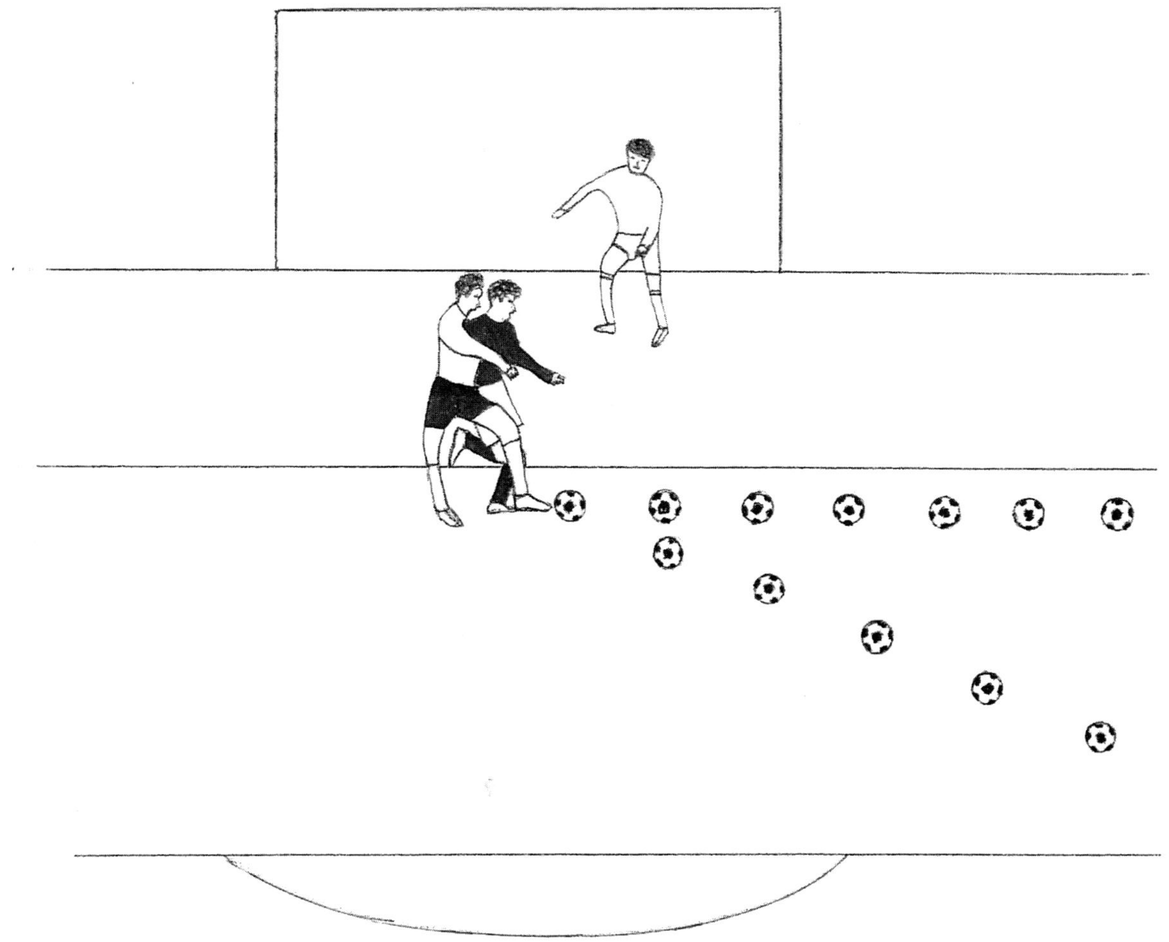

The Defining Moment in Defence in the Vertical Plane - in the air – Statutory, in-play

The leap velocity, and height of leap coupled with your head or foot clearance angles are essential. Where defending of the ball in the air is concerned the defender must get in front of the opponent – to get the ball first, and apply the following techniques to various defending situations. When a situation arises to defend – the defenders reaction and response are PROMPTED by the "QUEEN HORNET – QUEEN BEE" analogy to defend his / her goal area at all times – timing – leap velocity and height of leap a must.

In Fig 4 – 7 defending a corner kick, the defender is prompted to get in front of the opponent and to use an obtuse (nearer the 90 degrees angle) to get under the ball to send it safely over the bar for a corner.

In Fig. 5 – 7 defending an angled cross, the defender is prompted to get in front of the opponent, and to use an acute angled head flick to send the ball safely around the goalpost for a corner.

In Fig. 6 – 7 the defender is prompted to get in front of the opponent to use a foot clearance to send the ball safely away from his / her goal mouth for a corner.

In Fig. 7 – 7 defending a long throw, the defender is prompted to get in front of the opponent to use an obtuse angle (nearer the 90 degrees) to get his / her head under the ball similar to Fig. 4 – 7 to head the ball safely over the bar for a corner.

Sometimes the player will have to make a split second decision as to whether to send the ball for a corner kick or to save a corner kick and send the ball to another part of the pitch – but what he / she must not do, is to send the ball to an opponent – if you are not sure use safety first and put the ball safely out of play.

PROMPTED by the "QUEEN HORNET – QUEEN BEE" analogy to stop the ball from going into your net is the PRODUCTION of the DEFINING MOMENT IN DEFENCE in the horizontal and vertical planes.

Keeping a CLEAN SHEET against any opponent – especially a strong one is not easy – but it will become easier, with plenty of Perfect Practice, using the production of the DEFINING MOMENT IN DEFENCE in both the HORIZONTAL and VERTICAL PLANES.

The Defining Moment in the Defence in the Vertical Plane – in the Air – high corner kick Fig. 4 – 7 get in front of the opponent and clear safely over the bar using an obtuse angle (nearer the 90 degrees) head clearance, set-play.

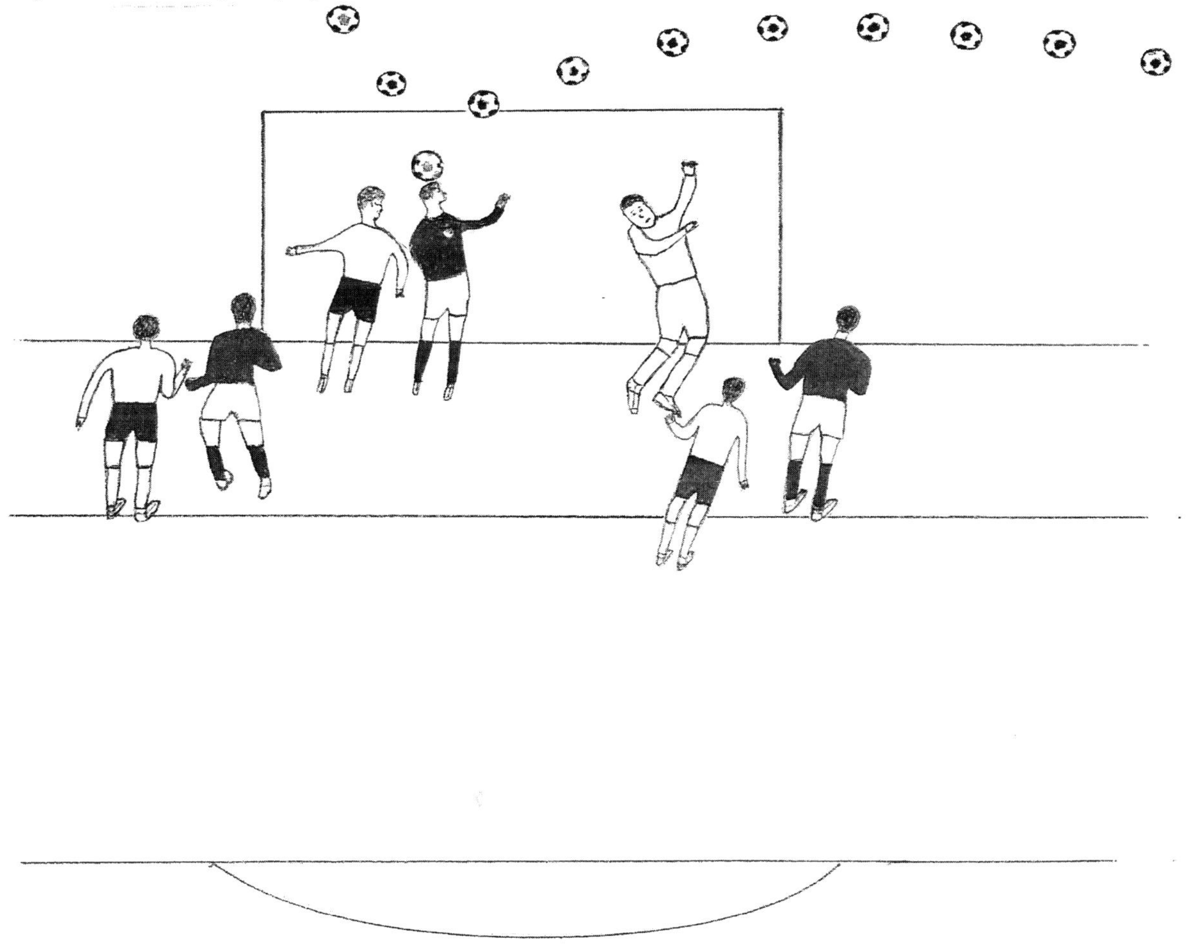

Perfect Practice the defining moment in defence in the vertical plane for IN-PLAY and SET-PLAYS
Perfect Practice the defining moment in defence in the horizontal plane for IN-PLAY and SET-PLAYS

To dispossess an opponent in the vertical plane – ball in the air – get in front of the opponent – get to the ball first and win it, Fig. 4 – 7 and Fig.5 – 7.
To dispossess an opponent in the horizontal plane – ball on the turf – get in front of the opponent – get to the ball first and win it, Fig.2 – 7 and Fig. 6 – 7. If the opponent has the ball at his / her feet you can quickly place your foot between the opponent foot and the ball and take the ball away – it's like placing a wedge between the ball and the opponent foot, except with more emphasis on winning and keeping the ball, rather than knocking over or causing injury to the opponent. Deliberate injury to an opponent is strictly prohibited.

Clearances

One important factor in defending under pressure is NO HESITATION head or foot clearance in general, and in dangerous areas in particular, whether you have to dispossess the opponent or if the ball falls to you, intercept a cross or a pass – the clearance must be made quickly, safely and with no hesitation.
Use safety first, if not sure.

Goal Line Clearance

If the goalkeeper loses his / her feet or is caught out of position, two or three, quick thinking defenders must position themselves on the goal line, to try to clear or stop the ball from going in – usually done during a set piece or free kick – then this could leave unmarked opponents free, not an easy choice.

Foot Clearance – vertical plane – in the air Fig. 6 – 7 low cross above the turf – get in front of the opponent with no hesitation foot clearance, to guide the ball to another part of the pitch, but not to an opponent or for a corner.

Defending an Angled Cross in the Tight Angled Corridor – vertical plane – in the air
Fig. 5 – 7 get in front of the opponent and depending on the height of the cross – if the cross is low use an acute flick to send the ball around the goalpost: if the cross is high and goal bound use an obtuse angle head clearance to safely send the ball over the bar as in Fig. 4 – 7, in-play

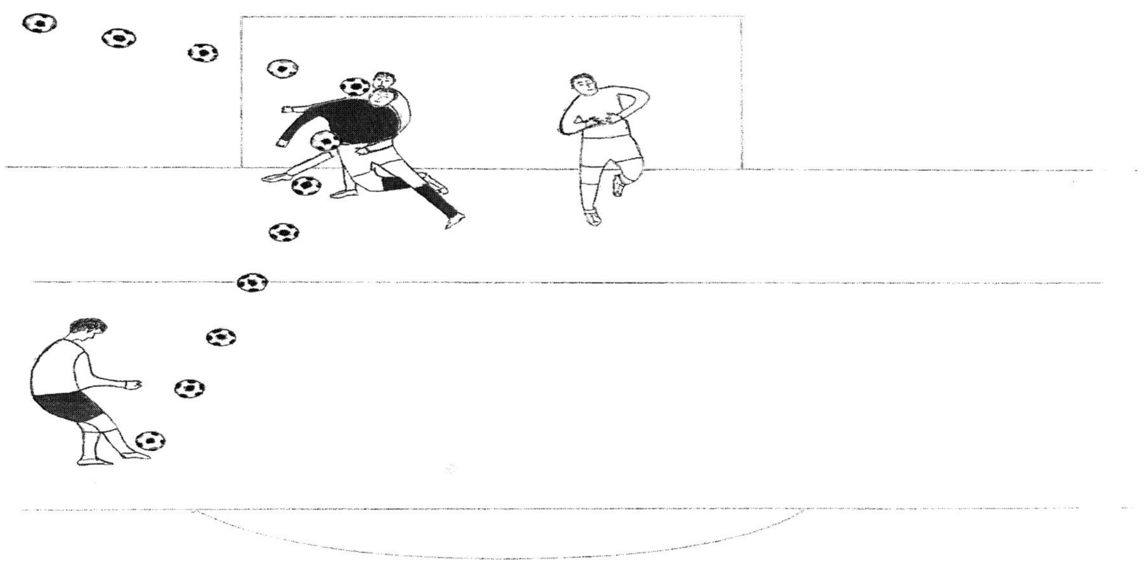

Foot Clearance – vertical plane – in the air Fig. 6 – 7 low cross above the turf – get in front of the opponent with no hesitation foot clearance, to guide the ball to another part of the pitch, but not to an opponent or for a corner, in-play.

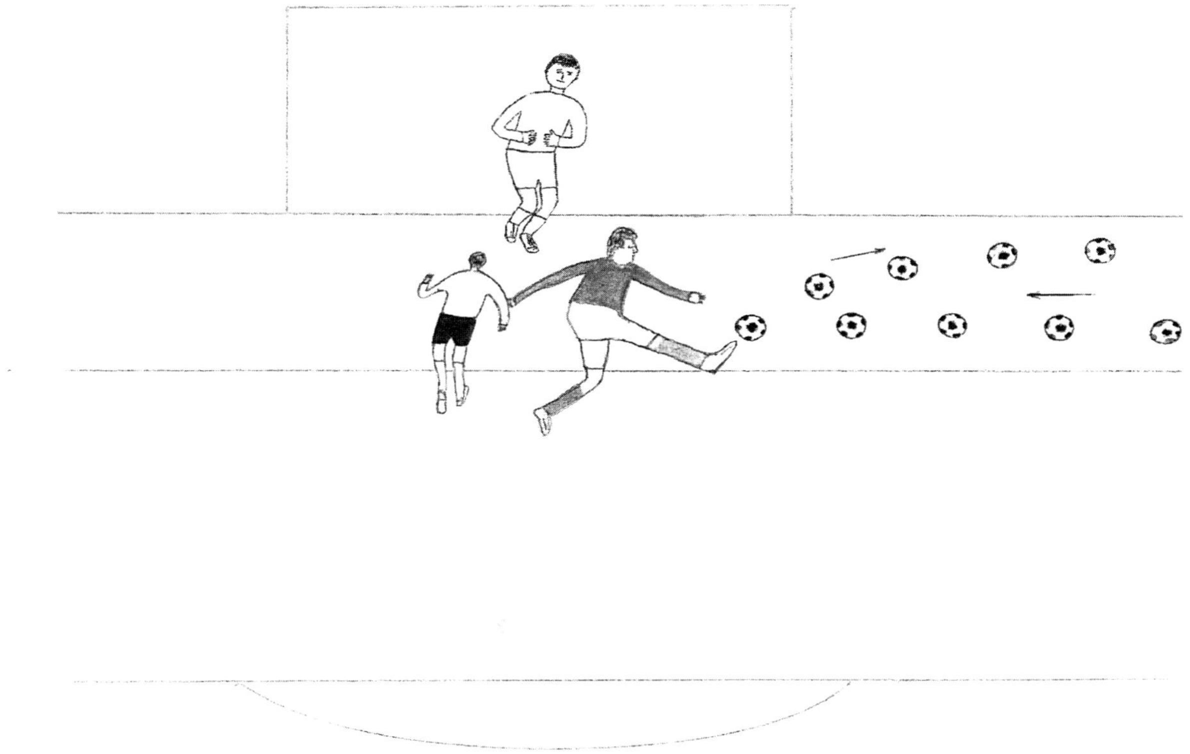

Interception – Closing Down – Tight Marking – Time and Space

For example, if an opposing winger moves down the flank with the ball, and delivers a slide rule on the turf pass or a pass that is about one metre off the turf or even head high to an unmarked team-mate and the ball is kicked with a velocity of $30\ m\ s^{-1}$: if the distance from the winger at the moment of striking the ball to his / her unmarked team-mate is 30 metres the ball would arrive at that team-mate in 1 second.

Assume your team-mates have maximum velocities of $8\ m\ s^{-1}$ to close down the unmarked opponent would require that your team-mates be in a position, so as to arrive in front of the opponent to block that opponent off before the ball arrives: this means that the closing down distance must be such that it should take slightly less than 1 second to reach the opponent – that is, if a team-mate is about to close down an opponent, he / she should be less than 8 metres away from the opponent to give yourself time – space and a chance to get in front of the opponent: to get to the ball first, in order to clear the ball or dispossess the opponent from danger areas - awareness, tight marking: reaction and response being prompted, are essential at all times. Some players have a better perception of time and space than others. Use mental judgement for 1second time lapse that is a period of 1 second, and 10yds / m for distances.

Ball watching by players – players must wipe out the thoughts of ball watching as a spectator from their memories during the game; do not become spectators on the pitch during the game, while team-mates are struggling to win the ball – know the difference between: when you are a player on the pitch, and when you are a spectator off it. Players should Perfect Practice switching from one to the next, as the occasion arises. Remember the defining moment in defence - in the horizontal and vertical planes.

Ball watching tends to have an hypnotic effect on the players for a moment or longer – and it is this time lapse which allows the opponent in with a chance to win the ball, gain possession, make a goal scoring pass, or score.
Ball watching reduces the players REACTION and RESPONSE TIMES.

A QUICK REACTION REQUIRES – A QUICK AND SAFE RESPONSE TIME WHEN DEFENDING.

Chances in Defence

Players must not give chances to the opponent – for example, poor clearances, a bad tackle, tackling from behind in dangerous areas or a bad pass or give the ball away to the opponent – lose the ball. Slow back-tracking and cannot get back in time to block off the opponents. Slow reaction and response time, ball watching, regular loss of possession – sitting back. Sloppy and careless defending must be avoided – waiting for the referee to blow the whistle; arguing with the referee and doing silly things that gets you sent off. Giving away unnecessary corners and free kicks; especially free kicks in dangerous areas.

Pushing, pulling opponents or diabolical infringement must not be attempted in any event.
Players must not forget their defending rules such as GETTING IN FRONT OF THE OPPONENTS.

Defending under pressure – requires composure; think before you act situation: this is where Perfect Practice on the training ground comes in: when players become tired, they tend to make mistakes more easily; and forget their defending rules and responsibilities. Perfect Practice on the training ground will put this right; so that on match days the players know exactly what to do, when a particular situation arises. Errors made on match days must be assessed and corrected on the training ground: errors must not be repeated.

When the Midfield Loses the Ball – Holding Back 2 must keep their positions

Back 3/4 at times, will have to use in position face to face defending, to dispossess the opponent – especially when the opponent threatens your 18 yd / penalty area. Holding position for any of these defenders may feel boring, because they are not involved up front at times – but these players are doing their jobs by stopping any quick breaks from the opponent: they are in the right position at the right time, and when they repel an attack by the opponent: that is their job.

Sometimes, it is necessary for one or two defenders to link up with the midfield or attack, and when this happens, then if, one goes up three stays back – that is with 4 at the back or if, one goes up two stays back – that is with 3 at the back – to protect the goal area and to block off the opponents when they break – not forgetting that some of the midfield players and strikers to back–track and help out the back 3 / 4

Defenders must not leave the back door wide open at any time during the game. A team player must never tackle an opponent from behind. Do not make wreck-less and senseless challenges, and tackles in your own 18 yd / penalty area – get the timing right, go for the ball and not the player.
Dangerous tackles must not be carried out on any opponent – even on the spur of the moment or retaliation – think, before you act.
Injury to defenders can cause problems in defence, and the coach is to make sure he / she has adequate cover to cope with any emergency, that may crop up from time to time – this means that other team-mates should have been through the Perfect Practice defending procedures, and up to the mark: to fill in the role left by the injured defender – so that team defence standard, is not affected in any way or form. When an opponent turns a defender; the defender must stay on his feet and disposes the opponent or use no hesitation safe foot clearance: do not give up when the defending chase is on.

Open Channels – the path of least resistance.

Defenders must keep an eye on open channels, and block off before the opponent could exploit them.

Back-Track

When defenders go forward or in attack, they must back-track quickly, and get back into position: so that they are in front of the opponents: and not behind them: good back-track is essential for good defending.

Backing-Off in-play

This requires common sense, and good timing – knowing when to put the tackle in to the win ball: without bringing down the opponent: especially in, and around your 18 yd / penalty area – keep your eyes on the ball: get the ball, and not the player, with well timed tackle. This defending procedure requires a lot of care, and any backing-off tackles should, preferably be done well outside your 18 yd / penalty area.

Defending Within Your Own 18 YD / Penalty Area

Defenders must possess a high standard of THOUGHT- CONFIDENCE – CARE – COMPOSURE – FINESSE – ORGANISATION – DISCIPLINE – and CONSISTENCY.

Defending Corners and Crosses set-play and in-play

Leap velocity, and height, coupled with head angle clearance.
This procedure requires tight marking: coupled with quick reaction and quick, safe response. Fig 4 –7
Good understanding between defenders and goalkeeper. Defenders must get IN FRONT of the opponents at all times and NEVER FORGET – to close down the unmarked opponents. To get the ball first: to clear with the head or foot, away from the opponent. If not sure use safety first – get rid of the ball to safety. Use a taller team-mate to mark a shorter opponent where possible; get the timing of leap velocity and height of leap just right to get the ball first. Never use a short team-mate to get in front of a taller opponent.
The timing of the leap determines, whether the defender is in control or not – win the ball or lose it. With good understanding, loud, and clear shout – the keeper should know when to come out to collect – punch clear or to stand his / her ground. Loud, clear, and decisive shouts between the goalkeeper and team-mates are essential, so that mix-ups do not occur.
Sometimes an opponent or two, may try to SNEAK IN UNMARKED, so defenders must watch out for and get in FRONT of them, close them down, block them off – and no FREE HEADERS should be given to the opponents. The goalkeeper should, also watch out for any UNMARKED OPPONENT, and see that they are properly marked or closed down. In defending corners – always try to get the ball safely away from your goal-mouth.

Defending Long Throws set-play

This is another way in which the opponent will try to get past your defence by going OVER THE TOP: watch out, and get IN FRONT of the opponents – block them off – and get to the ball first, Fig. 7 – 7.
Again tight marking, as with defending corners must be consistent and maintained. Use safety first – head or feet clearances, if not sure: tight marking and good timing are essential to get rid of the ball, safely out of dangerous areas such as the 18 yd / penalty area.

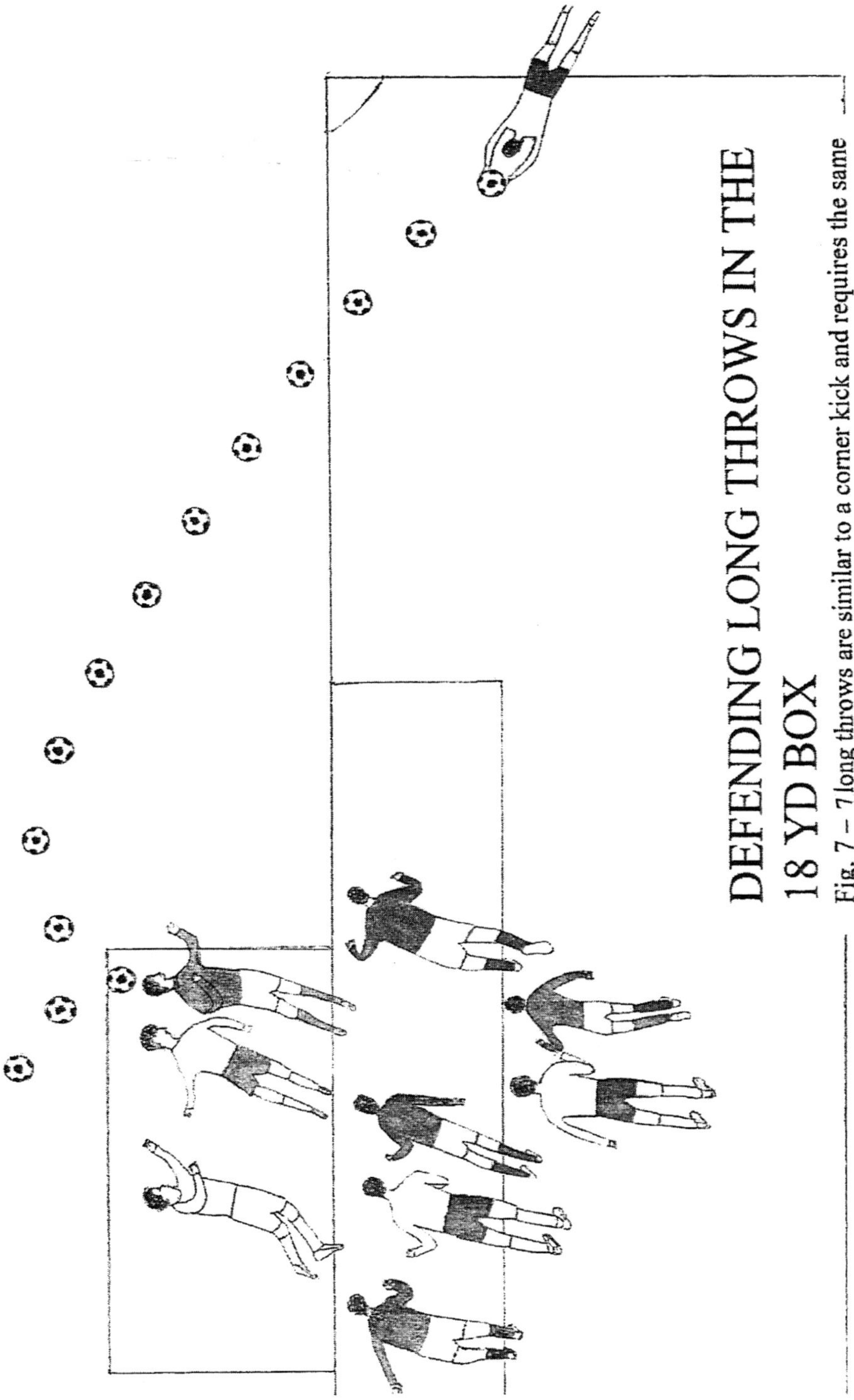

DEFENDING LONG THROWS IN THE 18 YD BOX

Fig. 7 – 7 long throws are similar to a corner kick and requires the same discipline as for a corner kick- get in front of the opponent, and use no hesitation obtuse angle head clearance to clear over the bar, or for a corner. The goalkeeper also has a say in this set up.

Defending Free Kicks Using a Wall set-play

Direct and indirect
Build the wall strong, and have it well organised in relation to the goalkeeper – the goalkeeper, should help to position the wall in such a way, so as to make the free kick more difficult for the opponent to carry out. Players must stand their ground, and must not create openings in the wall by moving apart or jumping upwards – there must be no weak links in the wall. Deny the opponent space.

Use good positioning of the wall, in relation to the goalkeeper; to make it more difficult for the opponent to break down or split the wall: make it difficult for the kicker to bend the ball, over or around the wall – so that the kicker has to alter his / her C.G – impact, miss the characteristic points on the boot and ball, and miss the target by over-hitting or under-hitting the strike.

As for indirect free kicks the opponent will try to spread the ball to make complete space – so the goalkeeper's reaction and response will have to be real good.

Direct Free Kick

Deny the opponent COMPLETE SPACE in both the horizontal, and vertical plane – defending a free kick; is like defending a long range penalty, with a wall between the keeper, and the opposing kicker. The minimum distance between the kicker and the wall is approximately 10 metres, Fig 8 – 7.
The opponent will try to kick the ball over the wall – through the wall – may get a deflection – and some cases around the wall. To stop the opponent from scoring, strict measures in the form of quick organisation and discipline must be taken.

For over the top – vertical plane: arrange the wall to be as close to the kicker as possible without breaking the minimum distance rule – so that the kicker has to alter his / her centre of gravity, by leaning backward: this will cause the kicker to increase the angle of elevation of the ball, and also, restrict the accuracy of the curved path ball – if he / she tries to bend the ball around the wall, in the vertical plane – the chances are the ball will go over the bar or miss the target altogether.

Defending a Direct Free Kick Using a Wall

Fig. 8 – 7 good keeper position – good wall to ball distance set up 10 metres. Kicker will find this set up difficult to score from - see curve path ball – the banana kick, under ball motion Chapter 5.

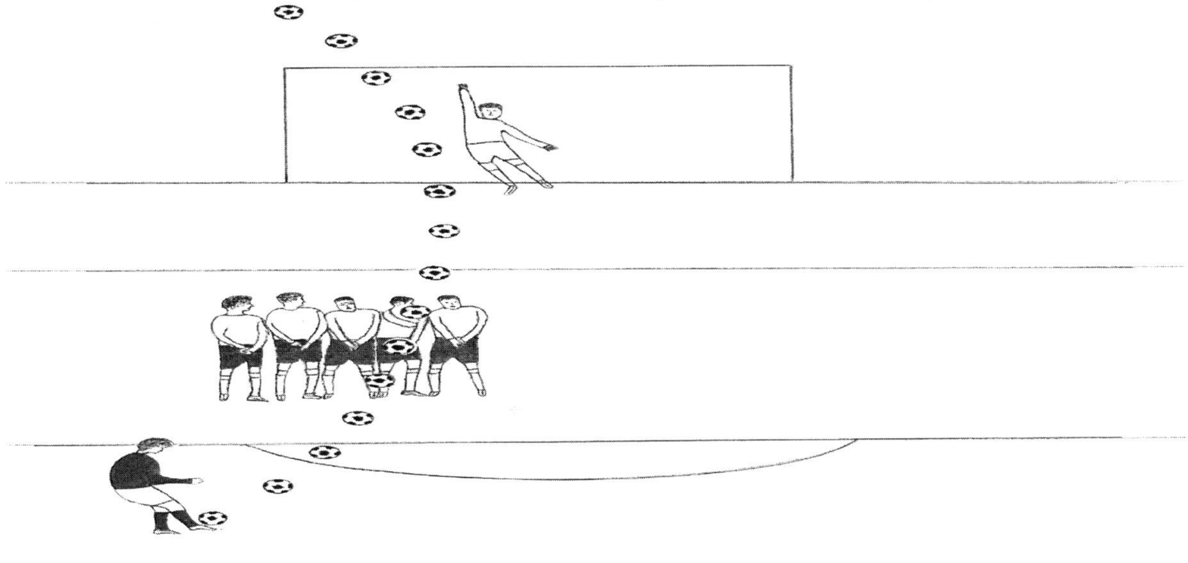

Indirect Free Kick – lateral thinking

An indirect free kick is more difficult to defend, because the opponents have an opportunity to spread the ball, and by-pass the wall – creating complete space before striking the ball toward goal: this does not give the defenders much time to close down the opponents, so good positioning, and agility of the keeper is required to keep the ball out: it can go either way; sometimes the opponents will score, and other times the keeper will save it.
The positions of the free kick on various parts of the pitch will have to be considered; and the wall intelligently organised in conjunction with the keeper.

Saving Penalties set-play

Saving penalties requires more luck than skill. It is quite difficult for the goalkeeper to know which side to go. As the word implies: it is a punishment: with a small chance in the keeper's favour to save, and a very big chance in the opponent favour to score – a good reason for players, not to commit a foul in the penalty area: go for the ball, and not the opponent.

Critical Times in Defending – Consolidation – Extremely Important - Remember

Defend for ninety minutes plus extra time – because there are CRITICAL TIMES during the ninety minutes plus extra time, that defenders become susceptible to lapse in concentration: this causes defenders to make mistakes in defending.

The times are:
First 10 minutes after kick off.
Last 10 minutes before half time.
Last 10 minutes before full time, and other times like when a goal is scored, and players get carried away with celebrating or when a referee blows his / her whistle for an infringement – so defenders must be aware of critical times during the game: and reassert themselves – be focused at all times.
Remember for defence, in-play, if you lose the ball – PROMPTER – win the ball back quickly.
Set-play, PROMPTER – get in front of the opponent to get to the ball first and safely away from your goal.
The KEY is not to give the ball away to the opponent at any time, if possible.

Chapter 8

Attack

Opening up Channels

Remember – when you are attacking – you are also defending, shielding, holding the ball, keeping possession, right down to creating chances, complete space, and control for the defining moment of the final ball. Attack the opponent, using the path of least resistance with the four dependent variables in Chapter 6. BE RAMPANT IN ATTACK.

1. Ball control
2. Passing
3. Possession
4. Final ball – THE DEFINING MOMENT OF THE FINAL BALL

There are two ways to attack the opponent in the horizontal and vertical plane.

DIRECT and INDIRECT

Direct

(a) Through the middle.
(b) Around the sides, and behind the back 3 / 4.
(c) Over the top, including long throws.
(d) Through a bad wall, from a direct free kick.

Indirect – lateral thinking

(e) Various angled cut back or pull back.
(f) Overhead kick.
(g) Back heel.
(h) Indirect free kick, deflection, disguised pass and long throw.

ATTACK - X NO - GO AREA

Fig. 1 – 8 when implementing the DEFINING MOMENT OF THE FINAL BALL – the player must remember that the ball is not allowed in the X "NO – GO" AREA and the goalkeeper's body area. The ball is only allowed to enter the COMPLETE SPACE area.

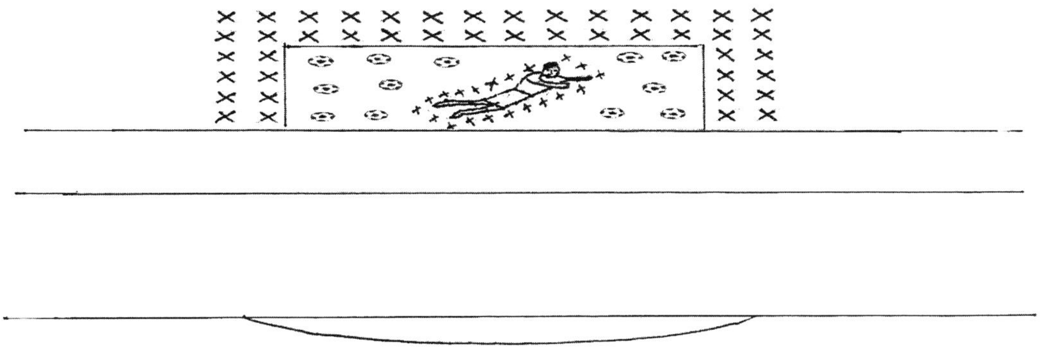

For attack – ball control, passing, possession and final ball must be at its optimum standard at all times – the players and coach should make sure the standard never drops – plenty of Perfect Practice.
Use side-foot slide rule fluent ONE TOUCH on the turf passes. Keep possession by putting together STRINGS OF UNBROKEN slide rule passes, right down to the final ball. Check levels of passing and ball control to see that poor control does not happen often – with a GOAL SCORING move in mind.

Pass the ball to your nearest team-mate and move forward, as you build the move: be careful not to carelessly give the ball away to the opponent – look up before you make a quality pass, so that the pass goes exactly to the selected team-mate, preferably an UNMARKED team-mate. Sometimes you have to pass and move quicker than the opponent as you see fit - to move the ball around quicker - the path of least resistance.

Use 80 to 90% on the turf passing and 20% long ball and high - ball passing, because long balls are harder to control and can often go astray – use it as an element of surprise pass.

The most important factor in ATTACK is to overcome, out–smart and out-play the opponent implementing the DEFINING MOMENT IN DEFENCE in the horizontal and vertical planes by implementing the DEFINING MOMENT OF THE FINAL BALL: in both planes.

Depending on the style you want to play by, for example, Chapter 10 – style 1 which is a more direct passing style or styles 2, 3 and 4 are more intricate, and indirect passing styles. The four dependent variables are also useful for other passing configurations, such as inter-passing and interchanging – and exchanging passes, from midfield to the opponent 18 yd / penalty area to split the opponent defence wide open.

Goal scoring moves will need Perfect Practice on the training ground. Make some of the goal scoring ideas STATUTORY- that is, these chosen moves with Perfect Practice week in week out, no matter what, and other goal scoring moves, should be added to the statutory ones, but should be changed from week, to week, to keep the OPPONENT GUESSING. The opponent will not be able to track you.
Use a good video - DVD to replicate moves or draw the moves on paper, and then put them into practice on the training ground; there are many great goal scoring moves to choose from – the coach will, also have ideas of great goal scoring moves that he / she would like to work out with the players on the training ground, and on match days to score some wonderful goals. There is no definitive number of goals that you can score, but as many as possible throughout the 90 minutes plus extra time of play, without letting in any goals will suffice – KEEP A CLEAN SHEET.

Some goal scoring moves from outside the opponent 18 yd / penalty area requires a co-ordinated attack – example 25 metre long range shot from a team–mate passing, and moving from the midfield area to score or an element of surprise strike to implement the DEFINING MOMENT OF THE FINAL BALL to a 25 metre strike, so that the ball bounces once, just short of the opponent keeper outside his / her reach, and into the net – there is a chance that the keeper may not be alert to the change in velocity of the ball caused by the bounce.

Specialist Task for Some Team Players in Attack

The coach or manager should know his / her best "SPECIALIST" players to carry out certain specialist task for his / her team. Some players may be good at more than one task, but best at a particular one. The dominant factor here is to use the player who is clearly the best for that task.
Like the team's "HOLD UP" player for example one with good tricky footwork, and close ball control to set up chances for team-mates in the box. Some examples in attack – in a set piece right side corner kick use the best player who can take a corner kick with slide rule accuracy to an UNMARKED team-mate in splendid isolation in the opponent 18 yd / penalty area: and the same for the left side.

Taking long range free kicks when the ball is still or running with the ball and striking from 20 to 30 metres from the opponent goal. Best at volleying in the opponent 18 yd / penalty area - and downward headers in the opponent 18 yd / penalty area etc., and players who are good at LONG THROWS.
If the players are equally good at different tasks – this is even better for the team – this gives the team more options and accuracy – and makes it more difficult for the opponents to cope with like using the "FASTEST DRIBBLER" to go past opponent with the ball.

These SPECIALIST tasks – for some players must be statutory, and have Perfect Practice.

Getting in front of the Opponent set-play and in-play

GETTING IN FRONT OF THE OPPONENT DOES NOT MEAN THAT THE OPPONENT IS TOO FAR BEHIND SO AS TO BECOME UNMARKED – IT MEANS CLOSE IN FRONT IN THE HORIZONTAL AND VERTICAL PLANES. GET TO THE BALL FIRST - FIRST IN EVERYTHING.

Team-Mate Surrounded by Two or Three Opponents in-play

Fig. 2 – 8, look up and pass quickly to your UNMARKED team-mate, and you must not try to be too clever, and hold on to the ball for longer than is necessary, and this applies to the "HOLD UP " player as well. Do not be selfish.

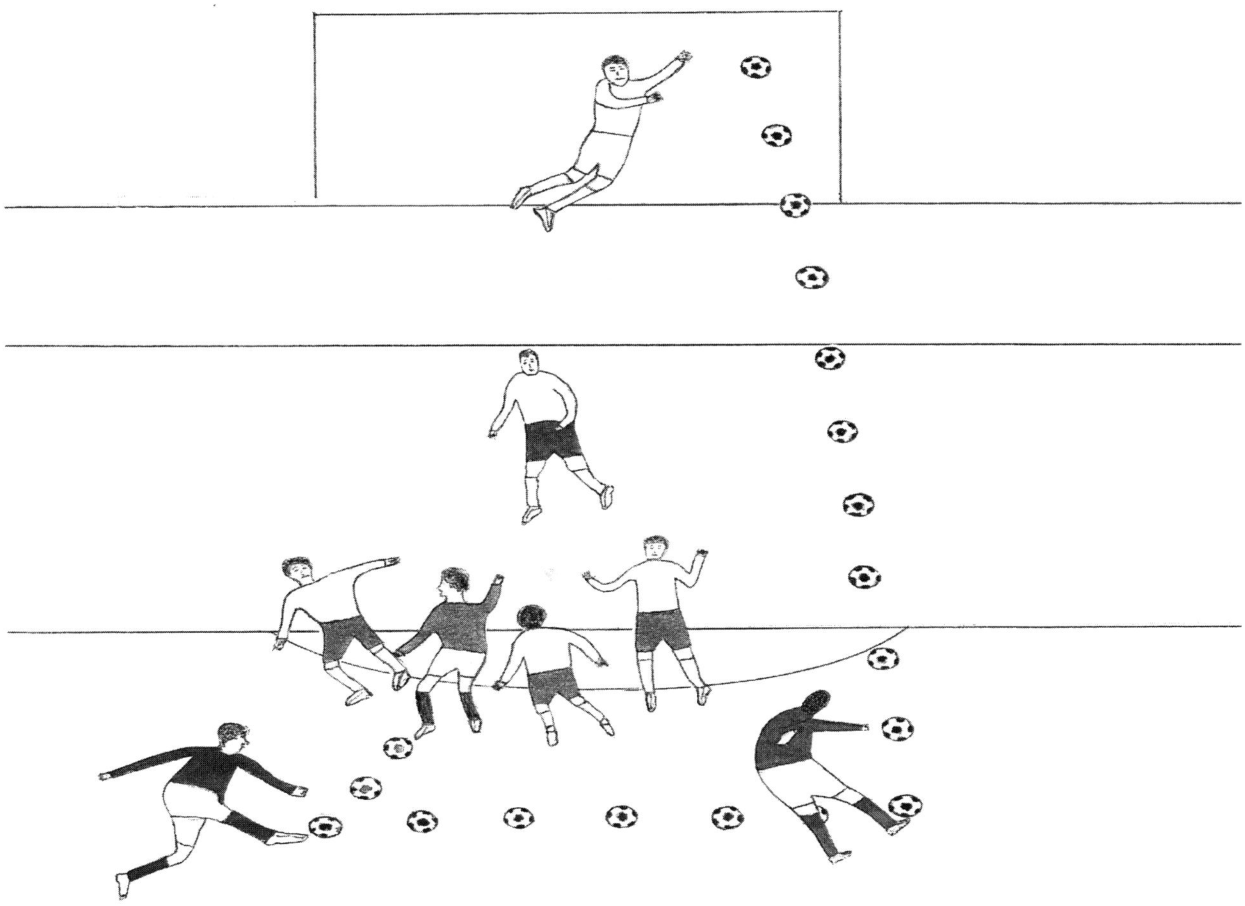

Using the Flanks - the path of least resistance

The wingers must use the flanks very often during the 90 minutes, plus extra time – to go past opposing defenders, and get their crosses, and passes into the opponent 18 yd / penalty area to the UNMARKED team - mate: use STATUTORY slide rule on the turf passes, across the face of the goal or crosses into the goal mouth – or varied angle CUT BACK into the opponent 18 yd / penalty area: supported by incoming strikers and midfield team–mates to implement the defining moment of the final ball: requires precision timing. Co-ordinate moves with team-mates and know exactly where some team-mates are, and where some should be.

Attack in Droves – Strength in Numbers

Attack with 80% force – that is, that two or three of the back 3 / 4 are always in position, and in front of the opponent to close down and block off any break or attack by the opponent: never leave the back wide open. Attacking in droves is essential for inter-passing, and interchanging in the opponent 18 yd / penalty using THE "HOLD UP" PLAYER or THE "FASTEST DRIBBLER"– the nucleus of the move.
The player who teases opposing defenders, and goalkeeper with his / her natural skills - the team's "Hold Up" player in the opponent 18 yd / penalty area – a naturally gifted player brave and full of tricks – such as good footwork and close control – to shield the ball – dummy opponents – send opponents the wrong way – to use fluent step-over when in possession and pursued by opponents – ride tackles – lay off chances, and half chances to the UNMARKED team-mate in splendid isolation – THE PROVIDER AND SCORER OF GOALS. Some teams may use more than one "HOLD UP" PLAYER – if one is heavily marked the other one will take over – switch from one to the next when things gets hot.

Running with the ball toward goal gives the player the impetus to accelerate faster than the opponent: but care is needed to give the ball the correct impact so that the ball does not accelerate faster than the player – too much impact and the player will lose possession or cause a break in play.

Turning Defenders

When you turn defenders – do it quickly, and decisively – the element of surprise.

Attacking Long Throws set-play

A long throw is another way of getting the ball over the top of the opponent defence – this is similar to an attacking corner kick: except the long throw is taken from the by-line by a team-mate using both arms and thrown from the back of his / her head, and with both feet on the ground – the ball is propelled over the top of the opponent defence. The force which is used to propel the ball varies from player to player – some players are able to throw the ball long distances, and into dangerous areas of the opponent 18 yd / penalty area, sometimes straight into the net which can cause a lot of problems for the opponent
When a ball throw is taken at mid-way of the pitch any player could take the throw – but when the throw is taken within the 18 yd line – the specialist long throw player should take the throw, Fig.3 – 8.

Attacking Overhead Kick Fig. 4 - 8 (a) –lateral thinking

This type of overhead kick is taken from an over the top pass made by a team-mate from any region of the pitch, and is usually directed at the opponent goal with a view to score – requires good skill, and timing to make it work: and of course Perfect Practice: an element of surprise attack.

Attacking Back Heels – lateral thinking

There are two types of back heels:

Normal Back Heel

1. Where a team-mate is in possession of the ball on the turf – except his / her own penalty area knows that a team-mate is close behind, and the back heel's the ball to that team-mate to either start another move or to score: this requires that the team-mate applies the correct inertia, and direction in order not to over-hit or under-hit or send it astray or to an opponent.
   NEVER BACK HEEL IN YOUR OWN 18 YD / PENALTY AREA.

Co-ordinated Back Heel – Fig. 5 –8

This is carried out in the opponent 18 yd / penalty area where team-mate number 4 is in possession with the ball on the turf in conjunction with team-mate number 2 following closely behind – when the team-mate number 4 with the ball reaches a certain distance outside the goal mouth - pull keeper - he / she accurately back heel's the ball to the following team-mate number 2 to implement the DEFINING MOMENT OF THE FINAL BALL. This move will have to be worked out with Perfect Practice on the training ground – again the correct inertia must be applied to the ball, so that the ball gets to the intended team-mate.

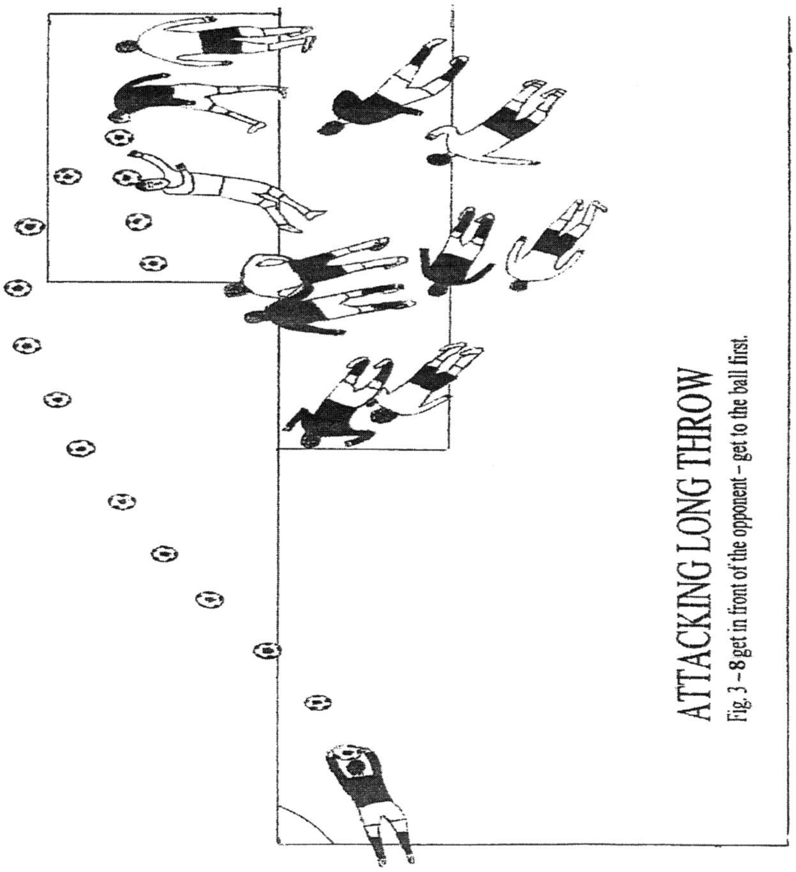

More Difficult Production of the Defining Moment of the Final Ball

The Overhead Kick Fig. 4 – 8(a) lateral thinking

Implementing the DEFINING MOMENT OF THE FINAL BALL for these two strikes requires that the player take extra care when learning and carrying out these strikes. The Perfect Practice must be carried out in the presence of a trained football / soccer player who is an expert in implementing these strikes, because of the extra number of factors, and an element of danger in the strikes.
Some players are naturally gifted, and these strikes comes natural to them - whereas some players will have to work at them to get the co-ordination right, and some players never get them right, no matter how much they try.
The stages required for the strikes are as follows-
First keep your eyes on the ball – a soft surface to cushion the fall – the kicking foot to kick the ball is on the turf, this foot helps you to defy gravitational force to give you lift off the turf as you leap upwards, the other foot is already on its way toward your chest, this foot helps to alter your body's centre of gravity to bring your body posture parallel to the turf, and facing upwards. As the ball approaches precise timing is required to get the leap velocity to the flight path of the ball - and the velocity of the kicking foot to match the velocity of the incoming ball, so that the foot gets behind the ball to strike it acutely downwards into the opponent net – almost at the same time after the kick is made, the other foot is automatically, and instinctively on its way down to the turf, followed by the kicking foot to help cushion the fall with the aid of both hands. All stages happen quickly and almost instantaneously when you get the idea right and the optimum standard is reached.

Sideways Scissors Kick Fig. 4 – 8(b) lateral thinking

The sideways scissors kick is similar to the overhead kick – except the body is turned sideways – that is, the side of the body is parallel to the turf when the strike is made. The lift off the turf, the change in body posture, timing the scissors action of the feet, acute angle, and complete space make these strikes much more difficult to carry out. These are spectacular strikes when they are done correctly. Do not concentrate on how spectacular the strike will look, but to get it right is more important.

Overhead Kick, in-play

Fig. 4 – 8 (a)

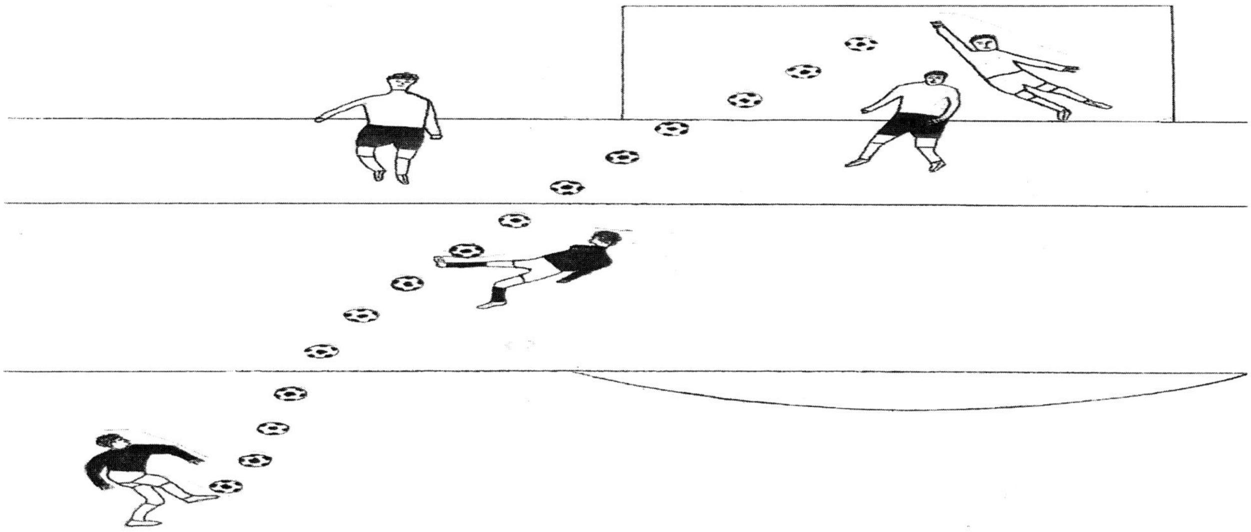

Sideways Scissors Kick – vertical plane Fig. 4 - 8 (b) slide rule cross from a team-mate in the tight angle area or corner flag to a team-mate in splendid isolation on the edge of the opponent 18 yd box to implement the DEFINING MOMENT OF THE FINAL BALL – lift off the turf, body posture and precise timing to meet the ball are essential for this special strike, in-play or set-play.

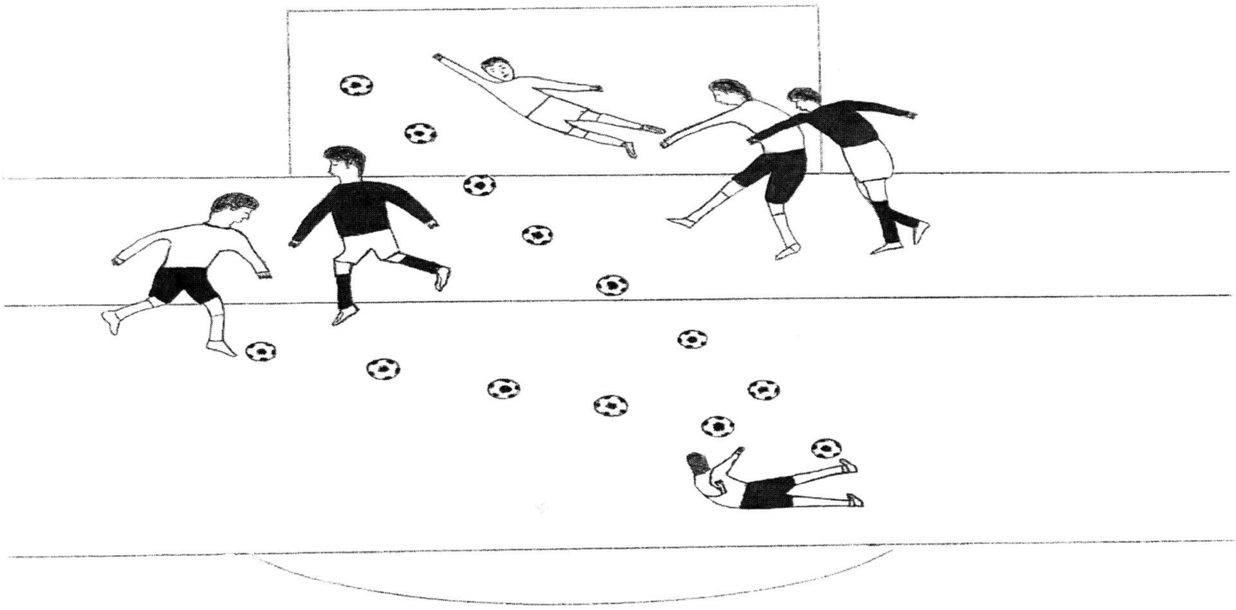

Co-ordinated Back Heel – pull the keeper to one side in-play
Fig. 5 – 8

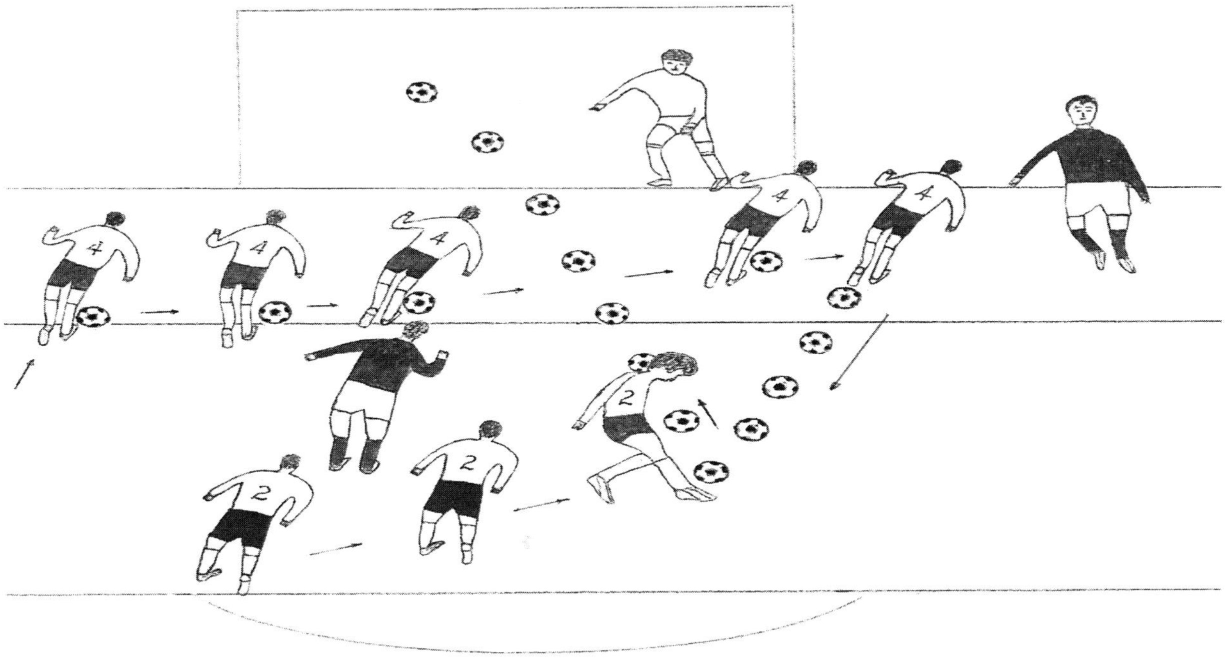

Varied Angle Cut Backs- Statutory Move Tight angle area Fig. 6 – 8

This move by the winger who gets into the opponent 18 yd / penalty area, and cut or pull the ball back with slide rule accuracy to an UNMARKED team-mate in splendid isolation in and around the opponent 18 yd / penalty area to implement the DEFINING MOMENT OF THE FINAL BALL, Fig. 7 – 8. Some goal scoring moves to be carried out in the opponent18 yd / penalty area requires a co-ordinated attack with at least two, or three team-mates in the box where at least one team-mate in total isolation is ready to latch on to the cross or pass to implement the DEFINING MOMENT OF THE FINAL BALL.

Ball across the Face of Goal – Statutory Move

Horizontal plane, Fig. 8 - 8 and Vertical plane, Fig. 9 – 8

This move is similar to the cut back or pull back from either winger, except the ball is driven parallel across the face of the opponent goal, to be latched on by a fast incoming forward team-mate to implement the DEFINING MOMENT OF THE FINAL BALL - if a ball is kicked by a winger so that it flashes across the face of the opponent goal for a team-mate to tap in: this requires good judgment of the incoming team-mate velocity with time in relation to release of the ball by the winger, as to what position of the goal mouth the tap in should occur – too far to one side of goal, and the ball could miss the target, because the ball will tend to maintain the velocity, and direction it originally possessed – Newton's first law of motion.
If possible the incoming team-mate ready to implement the tap in should give him / herself complete space, be in front of the opponent and make allowances for any skew in relation to the goal mouth to tap the ball in.

Tight Angle Area in-play

Fig. 6 – 8 horizontal plane

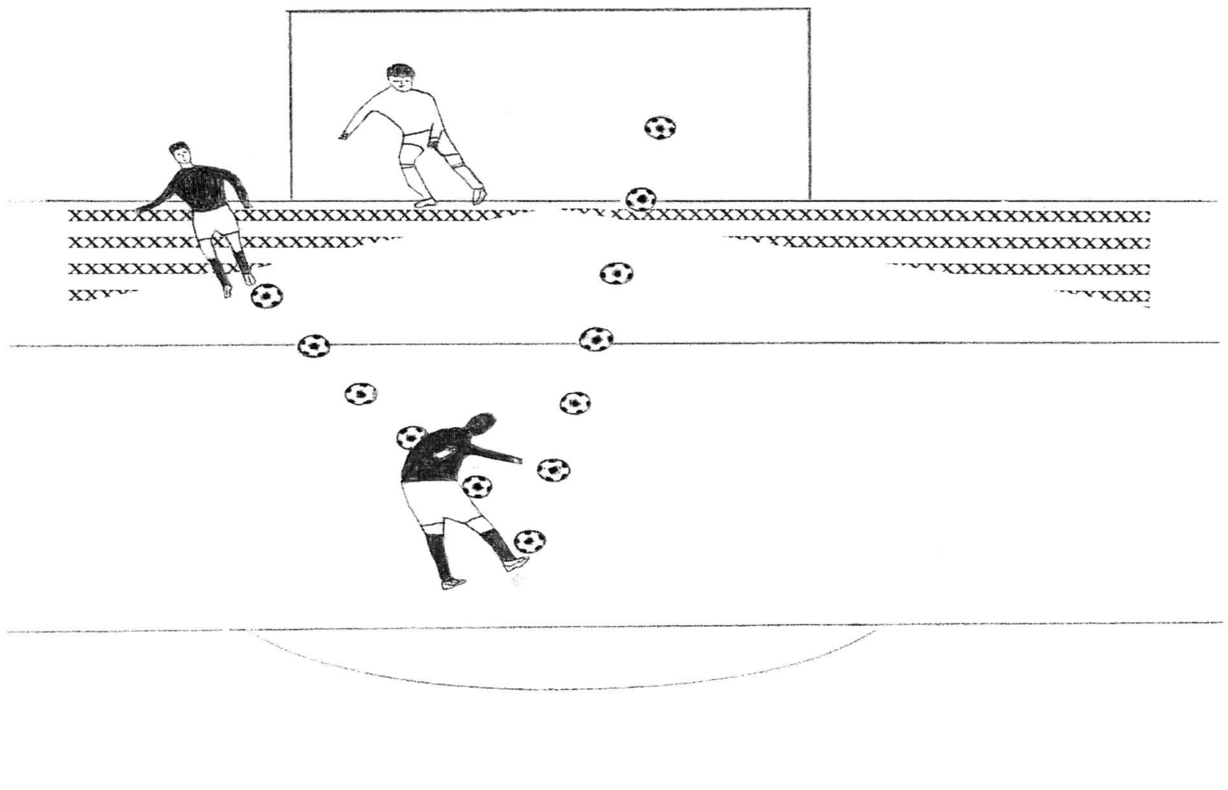

Cut Back or Pull Back - lateral thinking, in-play

FIG. 7 – 8

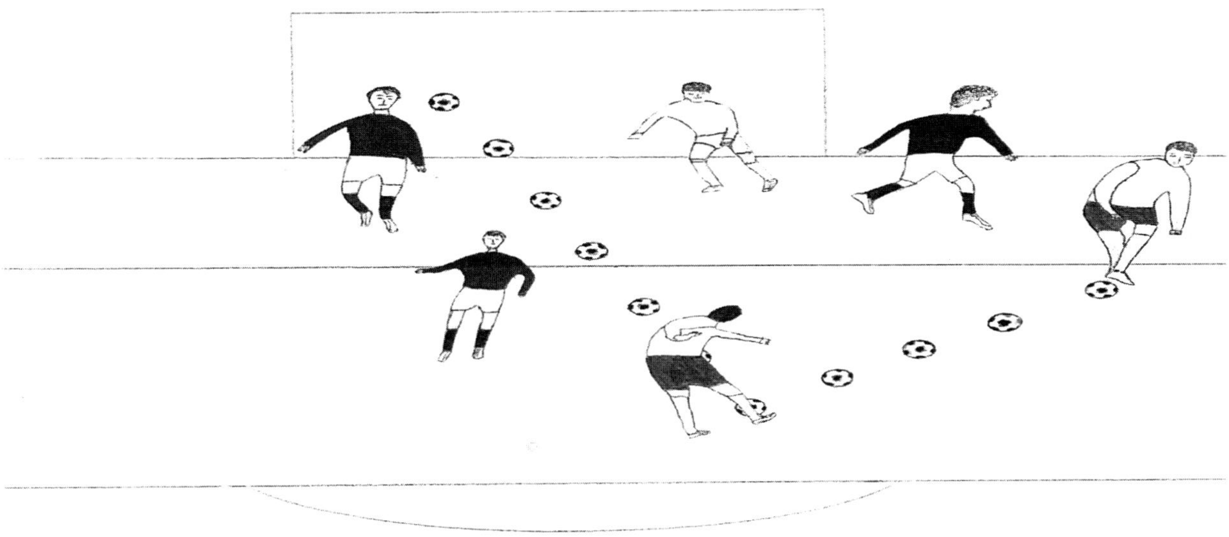

Ball across the Face Of Goal in the Horizontal Plane – on the turf Fig. 8 – 8 ball delivered by the winger across the face of goal – get in front of the opponent – be the one nearest the ball or get to the ball first – to guide, direct or tap in, in-play.

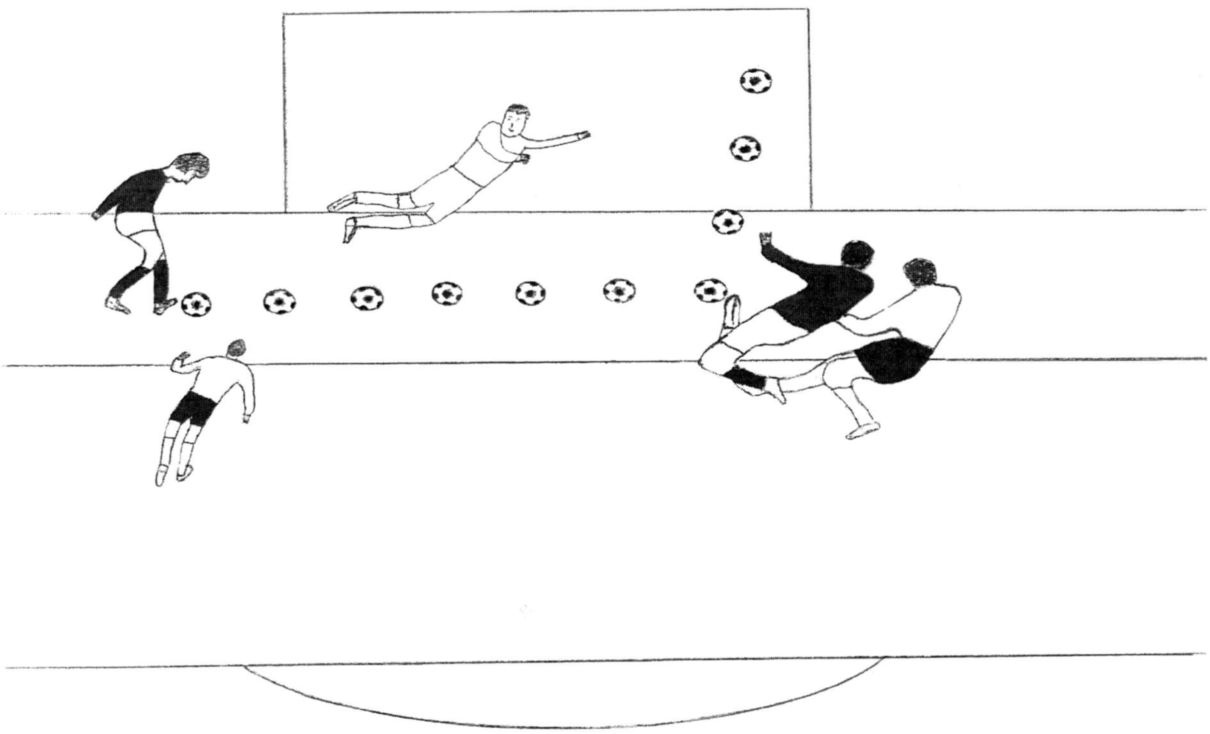

Ball across the Face of Goal in the Vertical Plane – in the air, in-play

Fig. 9 – 8 ball delivered by the winger across the face of goal – get in front of the opponent – be the one nearest the ball or get to the ball first to head into the net.

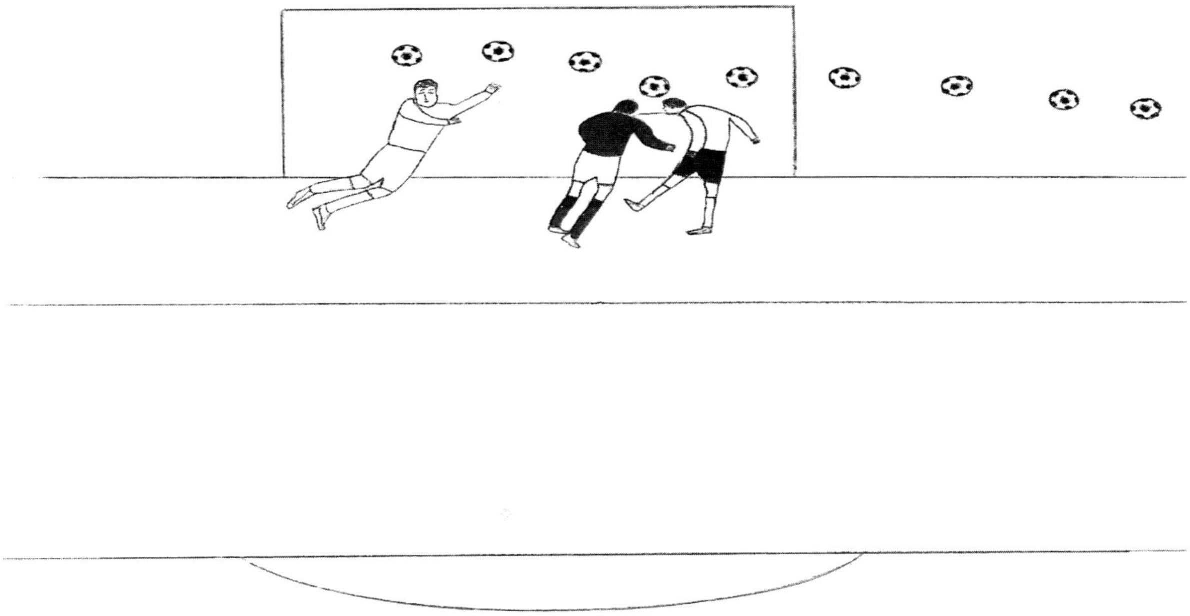

Attacking a Direct Free Kick using a Wall set-play

Fig. 10 – 8 bad keeper position - keeper off his / her line: bad wall to ball distance. The kicker has a good chance to score, and his / her reaction and response should be quick to spot any mistakes made by the opposing wall builder and goalkeeper – see curve path ball, under ball motion Chapter 5.

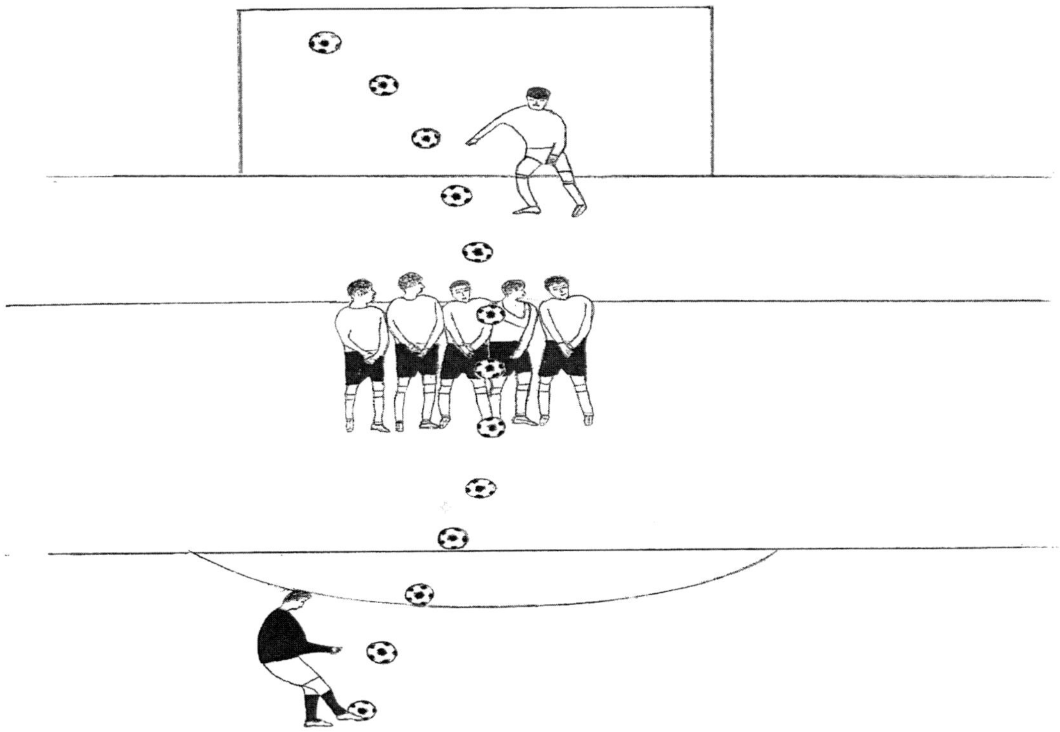

Pressing the Opponents

Keep pressing the opponents, and sooner or later they will crack.

Keep the Pressure up - do not forget - this is extremely important

Do not let the pressure drop – do not let the opponents off the hook- especially, **in the last 10 minutes of CRITICAL TIMES given**. Do what the opponents hate most, and turn up the heat. This makes them edgy, and nervous: it disturbs them mentally and physically: opponents tend to make mistakes more easily under pressure.
Attacking the opponents in their own 18 yd / penalty area require, a certain amount of – THOUGHT – CARE – CONFIDENCE – COMPOSURE – ORGANISATION – DISCIPLINE and FINESSE, AND THE DEFINING MOMENT OF THE FINAL BALL IN THE HORIZONTAL AND VERTICAL PLANES.

Celebration of Goals

Keep your discipline – only a few players to be involved in the celebration of goals: reassert yourselves quickly, and get back to being seriously focused – otherwise some hot shot opponent could seize possession, possibly score and spoil your celebration.

Body Language

When goals are hard to come by, players tend to show tiredness, lack of commitment, and become despondent – the opponents notice things like these, and raise their game – so do not show signs of weakness to the opponents: be fully focused mentally, and physically, for the 90 minutes plus extra time – remember your training ground Perfect Practice, and implement them.

Do not Waste Good Created Chances

When the opponent make a mistake – do not waste that chance – take advantage of it.

Do not kick the ball straight to the opposing keeper.

Do not kick the ball over the bar or wide of the posts.

Do not foul an opponent in the 18 yd /penalty area.

Do not make bad crosses and passes, especially where the final ball is concerned.

Aimless crosses, and passes, are ways of wasting good created chances.

Do not pass the ball to a team-mate who is in a worse striking position in the 18 yd / penalty area – especially where the final ball is concerned, and the angle is tight, and no complete space.

Lack of support in the opponent 18 yd / penalty area, is another way of wasting a good created chance.

Not implementing the production of the DEFINING MOMENT OF THE FINAL BALL fully is another good created chance wasted.

Not reacting to snap up chances, half chances, and rebounds.

Attacking Free Kicks set-play

There are two types of free kicks – DIRECT and INDIRECT

Direct Free Kick

There are three ways to attack a direct free kick.
1.Through the wall with a thunderous drive, straight-line or rectilinear motion.
2.Over the wall of players, and into the net past the opponent keeper - adjust centre of gravity of kicker to give the required angle of elevation or surface to air strike - the correct impact so as not to over-hit or under-hit the ball or to chip the keeper, if he / she is way off the goal line.
3.Around the side or over the wall, bend the ball so to speak – known by various names such as the banana kick – curve path ball – curvature – curvilinear motion – or space curve ball. See curve path ball Chapter 5. If the opponent build and place the wall correctly, with the help of the keeper, it will be quite difficult to score – but if the opponent, build the wall badly without much thought and nothing to do with the keeper, then there could be COMPLETE SPACE to explore and take advantage of: so this is a situation where you have to rely on the opponent to make mistakes in building and placing the wall Fig.10 – 8 and 11 – 8 and quick thinking.
Some opponent use more players to build a wall and some use less depending on the various positions of the free kick with mistakes or no mistakes.

Indirect free kick – lateral thinking

Taking an indirect free kick, you have the opportunity to by-pass the wall built by the opponent – this means that you can create COMPLETE SPACE to have a strike at goal by passing the ball to two or three team-mates lined up side by side – one team-mate stops the ball; momentarily, for the other team-mate to strike at goal. If the free kick occurred too far from the goal, then a forward possession move should be started, Fig.12 – 8.

Attacking a Direct Free Kick using a Wall set-play

Fig. 11 –8 bad keeper position – bad wall position, team-mates 1 and 2 makes dummy runs toward the ball in the opposite directions while team-mate 3 implements the DEFINING MOMENT OF THE FINAL BALL – using an on the turf or restricted angle of elevation strike. In this instance the ball is kept still before it is struck – note the complete space created.

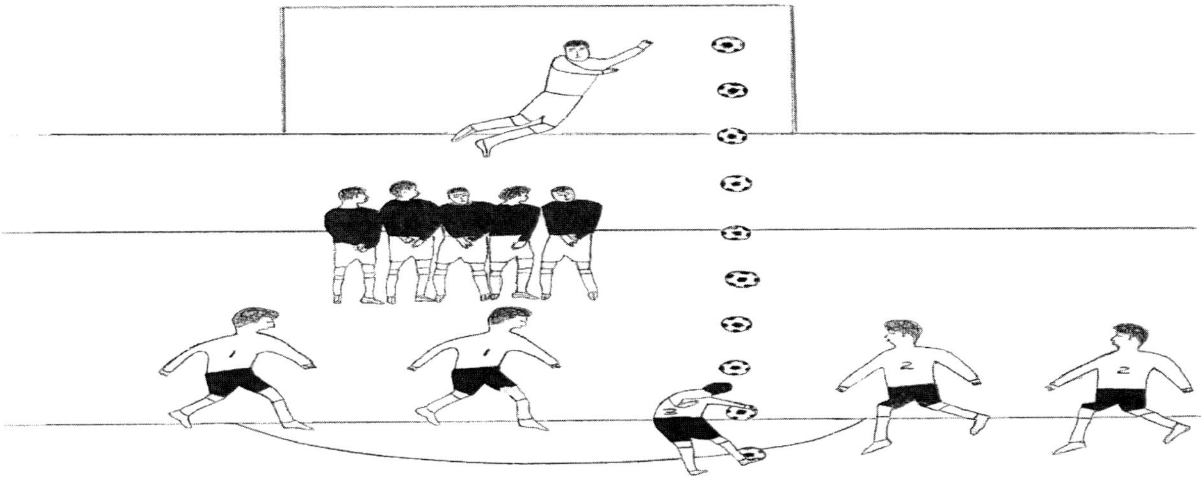

Attacking an Indirect Free Kick using a Wall set-play

Fig. 12 – 8 a good keeper-wall set up, but being an indirect free kick, team-mate 1 side-foot slide rule the ball to team-mates 2 and 3 who leaves the ball for team-mate 4 to implement the DEFINING MOMENT OF THE FINAL BALL using an on the turf or restricted angle of elevation strike. In this instance the ball is struck once to get it moving, then finally struck again – note the complete space created.

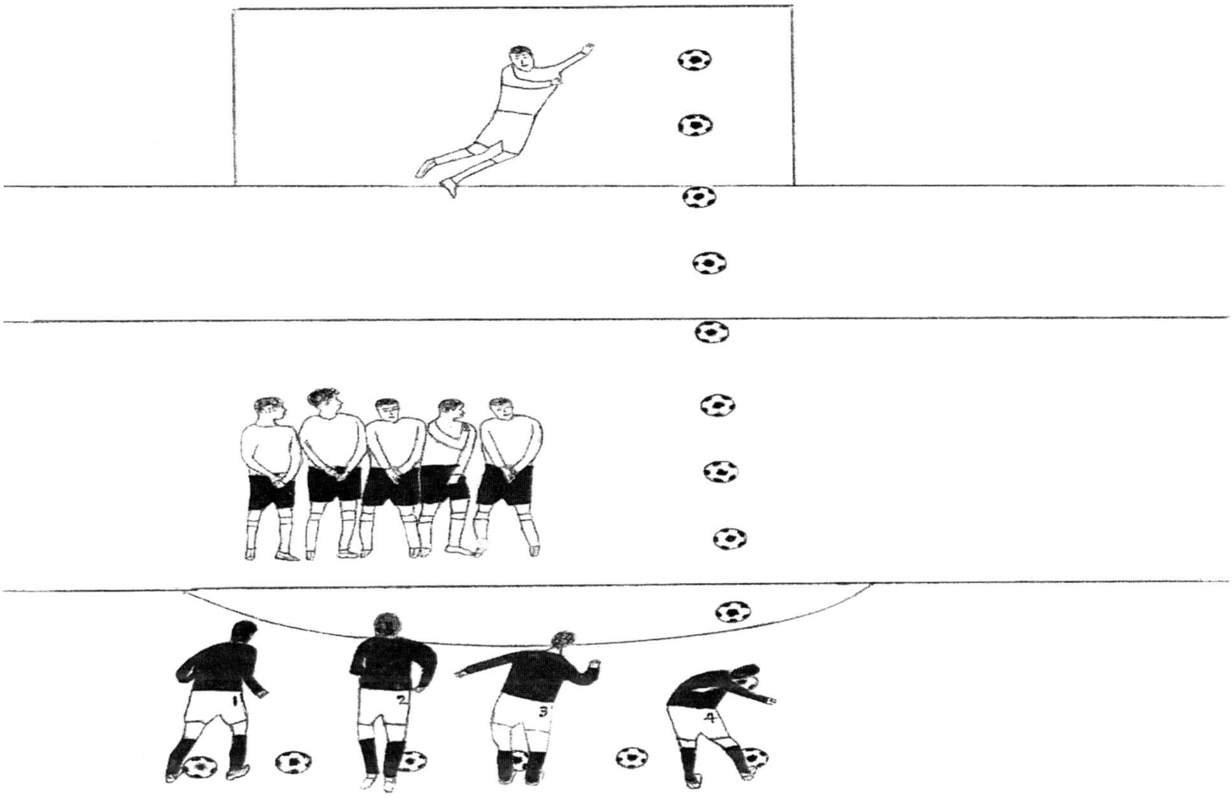

Attacking Corners set-play

Get in front of the opponent two team-mates dominates attention, while the UNMARKED team-mate gets to the ball first to implement the DEFINING MOMENT OF THE FINAL BALL.

Attacking corners can be done in the following ways. The most common ones are – where the slide rule ball comes in from the corner to the near or far post on to the head of a team-mate, to head downwards, for a scramble or downwards directly into goal – or for a knock back to an UNMARKED team-mate in total isolation in the opponent 18 yd / penalty area. Here timing and co-ordination between team-mates are essential to carry out this set piece.

The team-mate heading the ball must time his / her run precisely: so that when the ball arrives his / her leap velocity, and height, centre of gravity, angle of depression, and head velocity are such that he / she gets on top of the ball, at the moment of impact to direct it into the goal or to an UNMARKED team-mate lurking on the edge of the opponent 18 yd / penalty area – see Fig. 22 – 6 (a) (b) Chapter 6.

Other ways are: when a team-mate sneaks away from his / her marker to head the ball - a free header or use a cross from the corner to an UNMARKED team-mate lurking on the edge in splendid isolation of the opponent 18 yd / penalty area, to volley or sideways scissors the ball into the opponent net. Do not over-hit or under-hit the cross: keep your eyes on the ball and opponent at the same time Fig.13 – 8.

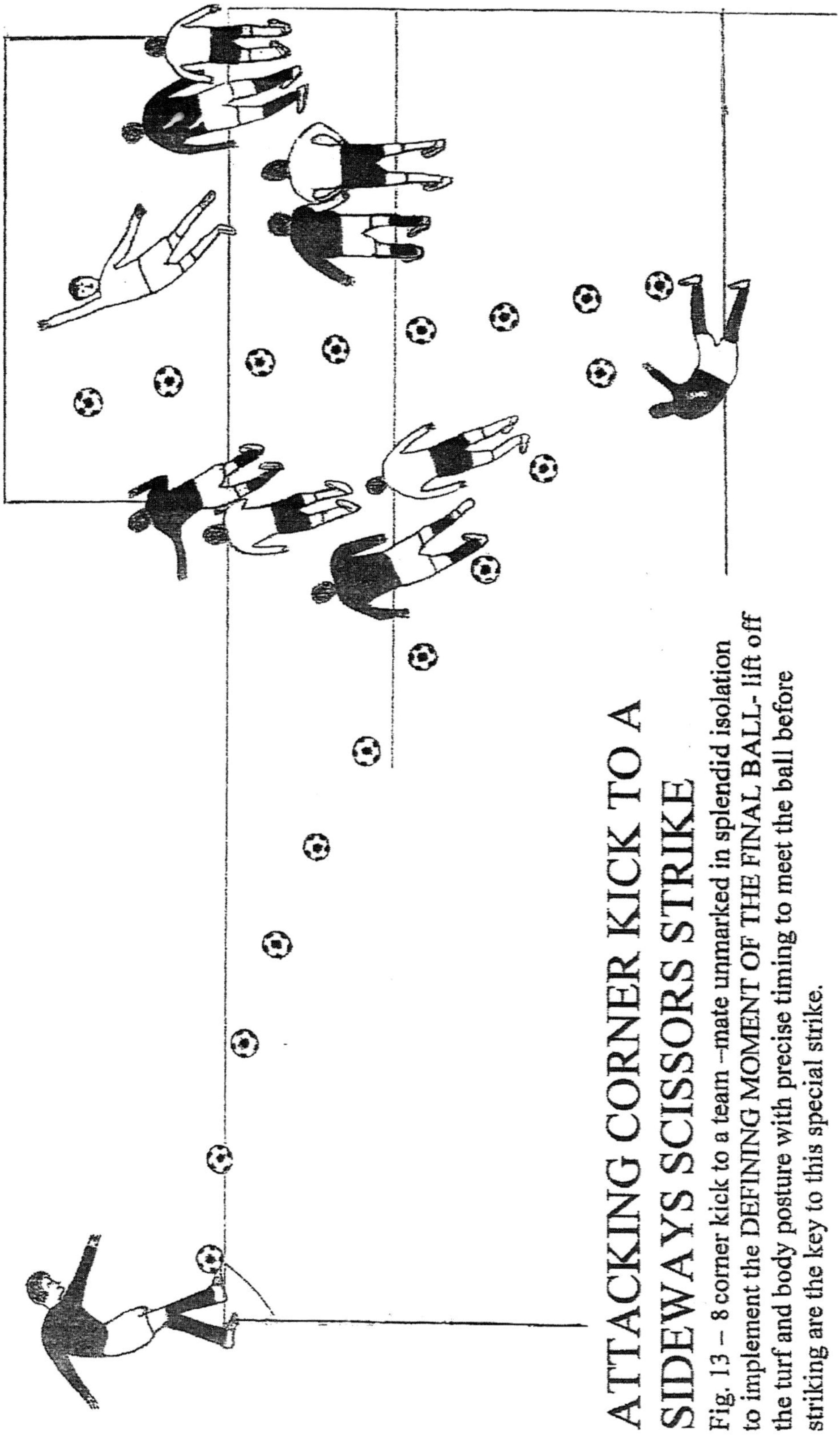

ATTACKING CORNER KICK TO A SIDEWAYS SCISSORS STRIKE

Fig. 13 – 8 corner kick to a team –mate unmarked in splendid isolation to implement the DEFINING MOMENT OF THE FINAL BALL- lift off the turf and body posture with precise timing to meet the ball before striking are the key to this special strike.

Taking Penalties set-play

This is an important aspect of the game, a punishment given to the opponent for committing a blatant foul in your penalty area – many results are decided by it. Penalty taking requires a lot of Perfect Practice, and ability to keep calm, with a cool head – mentally, able to block out the crowd, and their distractions: to keep your concentration and reduce the pressure.
Every player in the team should Perfect Practice taking penalties in training and should be able to score most times with a clinical finish. Be prepared and ready to take penalties, at any time during the game.

The aim is to put the ball past the opponent keeper, without too much hassle: and to do so, you first have to mentally confuse the keeper: you have to put an element of doubt into the keeper's mind, so that he / she does not know which side you are going to place the ball. The penalty kicker should know exactly, which side of the keeper he / she want to place the ball; and should be done in the following manner –

Look at the bottom right hand corner – get your control right – your centre of gravity – restricted angle of elevation, the lower the better; for penalty take. Remember your centre of gravity controls the angle of elevation – if you lean backwards too much when you strike the ball you will get underneath it and almost always you will kick the ball over the bar: you need to get your acute angle fixed in your mind – that is, from the penalty spot your acute angle will be your right side or the goalkeeper's left, and vice versa – use your safest kicking foot for the strike.
The acute angle, and restricted angle of elevation – is in the line of action of the force will help the kicker to keep the ball within the goalposts, and under the bar – once you are satisfied that you have every aspect under control, get your head down, and with the correct impact strike the ball into the left hand corner, Fig. 14 – 8 (b). The same principle can be applied to: look to the left hand corner strike the ball into the right hand corner, Fig. 15 – 8.
Sometimes the goalkeeper may guess the same side you want to place the ball; but there is nothing you can do about that – just strike the ball correctly, and hope for the best.

Ball Velocity and Keeper's Velocity with Respect to Time

Fig 14 – 8 (a)

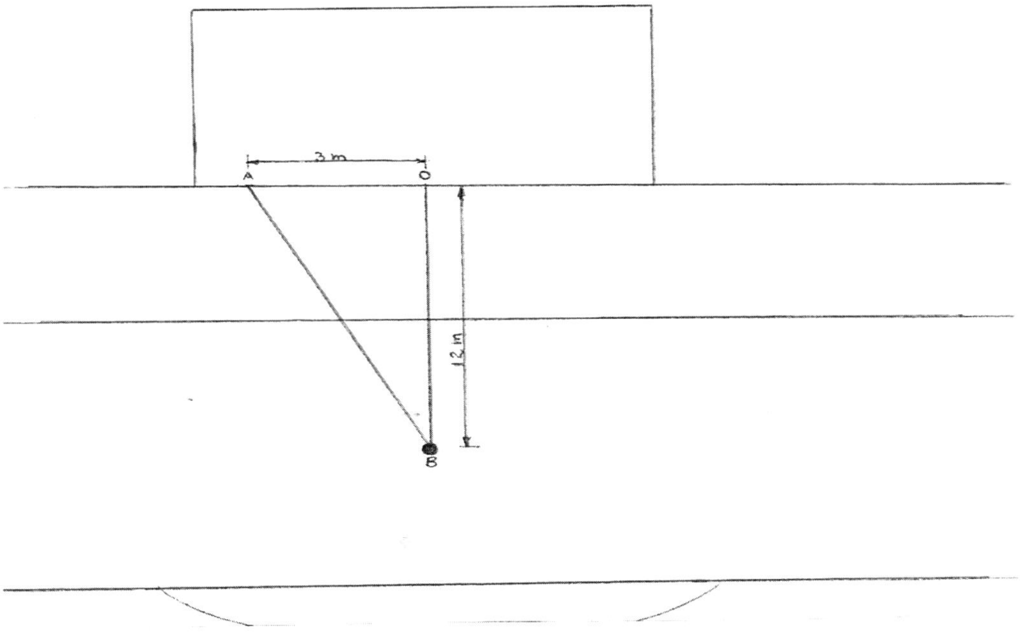

Assume the length of the goalkeeper with hands outstretched to 2.5 m, plus diving velocity depending on the reaction and response of the individual keeper. If the ball is struck at $30\ m\ s^{-1}$, by an opponent – the ball will take 0.4 s to reach the corner of the goal line – and if the goalkeeper can dive from point O to point A in 0.4 second or less – the goalkeeper has a chance of touching or pushing the ball around the post, Fig 14 – 8 (a)

Taking a Penalty set-play

Fig.14 – 8 (b) look right then strike left.

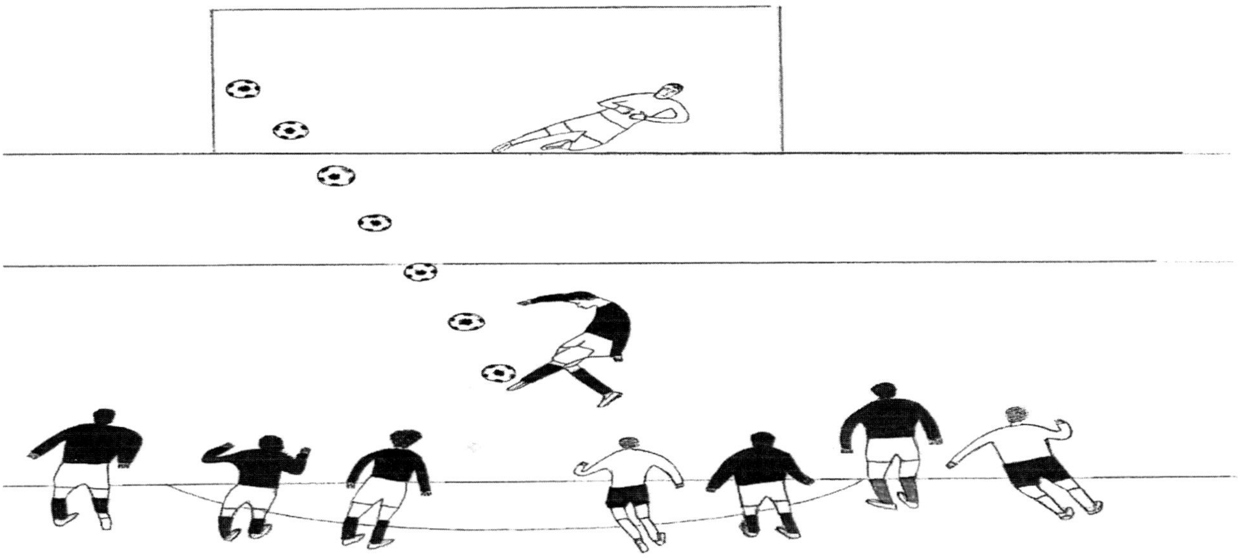

Taking a Penalty set-play

Fig. 15 – 8 look left then strike right.

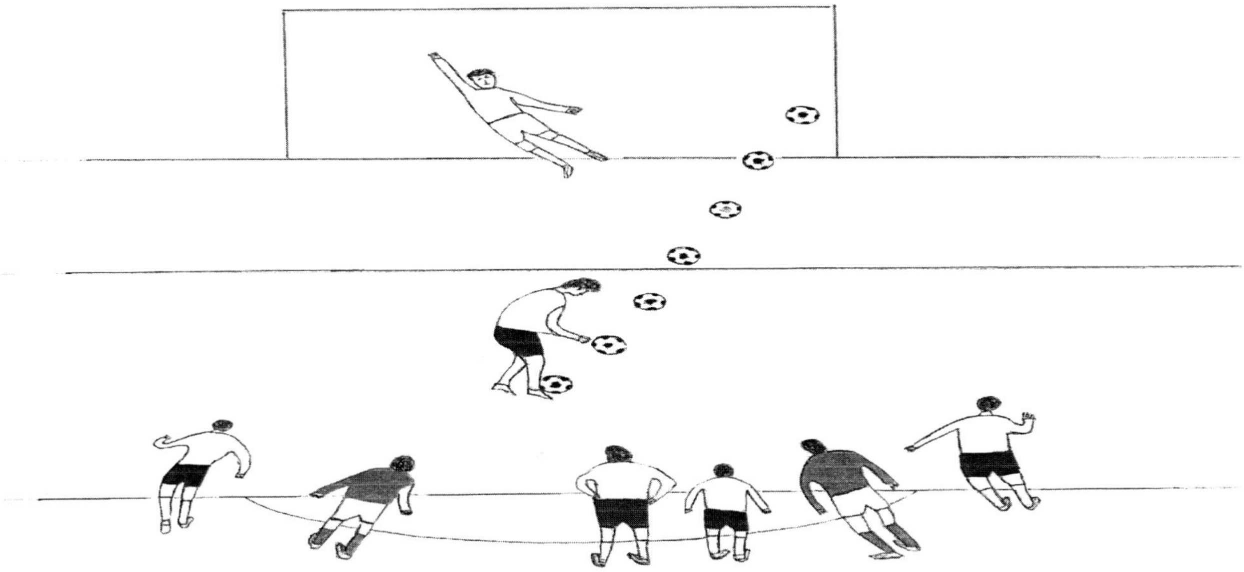

Training Ground Perfect Practices - Chapter by Chapter

When a car manufacturer designs a car, he / she develop the first one, which is the prototype. A lot of time, effort, energy, patience and finance goes into developing the prototype to get all aspects right. The designers Perfect Practice the theory before they put it into practice – they call it pragmatism. They use the prototype to iron out any mistakes or problems before the car goes on the road: in order that all parts are working in perfect harmony with each other: and this same principle is applied to football on the training ground. The training ground is an important department of a footballer's armoury: it is the place where all Perfect Practices are carried out, corrected and implemented – both mental and physical. The coach or manager should be in close proximity with the players to watch very closely: to point out mistakes made by players: and make the necessary corrections to the players and team to put things right before a game.

Health and Fitness as Chapter 1

Diet, strength, stamina, velocity and acceleration build up – this is where the club's doctor, physiotherapist, dietician, coaches and players self discipline comes in: so essential to the players for playing ninety minutes plus extra time – health and fitness are two things the players must get right before training starts.

Footwear

Footwear should be appropriate to weather conditions – so players know exactly what boots to wear on a dry day or wet day. Whatever boots the players Perfect Practice, their training in - should be used for playing and vice-versa – this keeps touch and contact with the ball to a consistent high standard in training and playing.

Training Ground Surface

The training ground surface should be comparable to that of the match day playing surface – smooth and grass length short: to keep ball control, passing, possession and final ball consistent. Playing surfaces varies from club to club – and players will have to allow for this inconsistency.

Mental Training

Players able to remember under pressure instructions from the coach and manual – how to keep focused on the Perfect Practice training and to implement the training on match days: and not be swayed by the opponent or other distractions: to show character to come back when things go wrong, by not allowing the Perfect Practice to leave the players thoughts at any time during the game. Mental training goes together with physical training – one cannot do without the other.

Back 3 / 4 – midfield players and strikers need to remember their mental and physical responsibilities. All team players to Perfect Practice the art of defence in general. The goalkeeper must remember his / her mental and physical responsibilities, correct elementary errors, such as dropping the ball when an opponent makes a fierce drive or otherwise. The goalkeeper must learn to cushion the incoming ball to remove its kinetic energy at the moment of contact from a direct drive - roll the ball out to team-mates. Do not give possession back to the opponent. Help to organise and discipline the back 3/4, to keep them on their toes – to keep the opponent out, a combined effort and a high standard is required by all: the coach or manager must make sure the standard of preparation does not drop below its optimum level.

Offside Trap

During training and playing, do not play the offside trap to the opponent – close down the opponent instantly instead, if you rely on the linesman for a decision you may get caught, because the linesman may not always get decisions right.

Clothing

Clothing and footwear worn by the players during training and playing should be streamlined and comfortable, so as to reduce drag resistance – and to increase the velocity and acceleration of the players during training and playing. On very cold days warmer clothing may be worn during training and playing. Baggy clothing and the wrong footwear tend to act like a small parachute – like the ones that slows down some aeroplanes when landing.

Training Ground Discussions

Discussions between coach and players, as regards to defending and attacking moves: and the understanding between themselves, giving, taking, remembering and obeying constructive ideas, in order to know exactly what each team-mate is doing or going to do during training and playing – awareness – anticipation – reaction and response.

Example – for an attacking move:
Two or more forwards with other team- mates and the coach, and says this is what we will do, and we expect you guys to be in certain UNMARKED positions, so that one of us will look up and cross or pass the ball to you and give us some well timed support so that you could implement the DEFINING MOMENT OF THE FINAL BALL TO SCORE.
The right wing team-mate says he / she wants the ball, so that he / she could run down the flank with it, then says he / she wants 3 or 4 team-mates to make well timed runs into the opponent 18 yd / penalty area. The winger says when the moment or signal is right he / she will release the cross pass or cut back to one of his / her UNMARKED team-mates in splendid isolation, to implement the DEFINING MOMENT OF THE FINAL BALL to score by heading, side-footing or volleying past the opponent keeper.

Occasional decoy runs by either flank players without the ball being passed to him / her momentarily – then the ball is released, so that the decoy player could exchange passes with his / her team-mates or go on to score.
So work out the theory – discuss it amongst your selves, make sure all players knows exactly what they suppose to do and this includes the goalkeeper, then Perfect Practice the moves on the training ground, using 11 a side till you get it right – keep it right, and implement the moves on match days.

Some moves are statutory, and must be done automatically and instinctively. Different additional moves must be added to the statutory ones, and additional moves should be replaced by new additional moves, from match to match, and from week to week – this keeps the opponents guessing and makes it more difficult for the opponents to know what you are going to do next.

Training and playing go together – one cannot do without the other, so when you train, you do it well, when you play, you do it well and then extend the training into playing on match days. START POINT-

Before you start training, get your doctor to give you a medical to make sure there are no serious health problems. Get your health and fitness up to a good standard – then work at it to keep it up – healthy diet and the appropriate exercises. Gradual build-up of – strength – stamina – velocity – acceleration and retardation, leap velocity – change of direction with and without the ball – these are a must.

Choose one of the styles given in Chapter 10 and – Perfect Practice complete ball control – passing – possession, and the DEFINING MOMENT OF THE FINAL BALL in Chapter 6.
The standard of these four variables must be of the highest quality or faultless – the tools for defence and attack.
Then go on to DEFENCE as given in Chapter 7. When you are satisfied that your defence is leak proof, then go on to, ATTACK as given in Chapter 8.
Styles 1-2-3 and 4 contain some good goal scoring moves, some statutory, some additional – and Prefect Practice required. A good goal scoring video/DVD should be used in addition to the given moves – the coach's experience and ideas must also come in to it.
Use 11 a side in training to look for, and iron out mistakes. This is the time to make corrections. Mistakes will happen, but with Perfect Practice they will be reduced to a minimum.
All problems mental and physical must be sorted out on the training ground and before every game. Sometimes it will be necessary for the coach or manager to keep on at the players to put things right during the game, because under pressure, players tend to forget their responsibilities and make mistakes more easily.
Remember in defence, if one or two back 3/4 goes forward to link up with the attack – two or three defenders always stays back in position to be in front of the opponents at all times during the game – to close down and block off any quick breaks by the opponent.

On the training ground IN THE FIRST 45 MINUTES PLUS EXTRA TIME score a goal or two with a clean sheet - the first half is done- then IN THE SECOND 45 MINUTES PLUS EXTRA TIME score a goal or two with a clean sheet – transfer this way of playing to match day games – home and away - job is well done.
The goalkeeper, back 3/4 midfield players and strikers to discuss – work out, for example, if a left back goes forward to link up with the attack – a left sided midfield team-mate who is good with both feet will move into the vacant left back position automatically and instinctively – or the goalkeeper who is in a good position notices gaps and call upon his / her midfield team-mates to back-track, and fill the gaps.
MENTAL JUDGEMENT use 10yd / m for working out distances – find out period for 1 sec time lapse - for velocity use distance with respect to time – and for angles learn all the common different angles and triangles and when to implement them.

Remember in defence LOOK OUT FOR AND CLOSE DOWN THE UNMARKED OPPONENT QUICKLY AND DECISIVELY DO NOT GIVE THE OPPONENT TIME AND SPACE – AND NO HALF MEASURES. Finish the job – keep a clean sheet - score as many goals as possible, and keep the ball in the opponent's half for the last 10 minutes plus extra time of the game.

Chapter 10

Match Day Kick Off

Four beautiful styles to choose – Train and play from.
These Styles are Extensions of Training Ground Perfect Practice.

The coach or manager should choose which style he / she wants the team to train and play from – and carry out the necessary training ground Perfect Practices, as described throughout this manual.

Style 1 – Quick – Direct

Consisting of side-foot slide rule on the turf, fluent, silky smooth one touch unbroken well timed passes: a more direct system to the opponent 18 yd / penalty area – using TWO TRICKY FLYING WINGERS.
From the moment of kick off on the centre circle pass to the right midfield team-mate who then passes to the winger – the right back, central defenders and left back must stay in their positions to defend their goal, goalkeeper and goal area for 90 minutes plus extra time: remember – the "QUEEN HORNET" and "QUEEN BEE" analogy – the DEFINING MOMENT IN DEFENCE – to keep a clean sheet. If you use 3 / 4 defenders at the back – as play is pushed forward, one or two defenders may move forward to link up with the attack – while one or two midfield team- mates fast back-track to fill the gaps left by the forward moving back 3 / 4 team-mates, the reason is, if you lose the ball and there is a quick break by the opponents, the two defending team-mates of the back 3 / 4 should be able to hold the fort till help arrives in the form of other defending team-mates, to close down, dispossess, clear or block off the opponents. Intelligent fast back-track, quick reaction and response are a must.
If at any time you happen to lose the ball during play – implement the DEFINING MOMENT IN DEFENCE, and win the ball back and start a move again. Bring Perfect Practice for set pieces into play when – and where necessary during the 90 minutes plus extra time of the game.
Pass, and move and ride tackles quicker than the opponent with a goal scoring move in mind – but you must also close down quicker than the opponent – STATUTORY.

Intelligent link-up play with forward team-mates, assuming the right back is in possession with the ball – look for the path of least resistance or open channel, and use side-foot, slide rule on the turf fluent, silky smooth, one touch, unbroken, well timed passes to UNMARKED team-mates: look up and pass the ball to a midfield team-mate or directly to the right winger or left winger, pass and move, accelerate or decelerate as the player see fit. The winger using the flanks very often runs at opponents, dribbling past them – holding, shielding the ball making sure well timed UNMARKED support have arrived in the opponent 18 yd / penalty area: the winger then looks up before he / she delivers a cross or a pass across the face of the opponent goal. TIMING and VELOCITY between the winger and his / her support team-mates to be spot on – too early or too late, and a good created chance is wasted. Once the chance to score has been created by the winger, the UNMARKED team-mate, should then convert the chance by implementing the DEFINING MOMENT OF THE FINAL BALL – with the feet or head past the opponent keeper.

The slide rule crosses and passes could be parallel to the face of the opponent goal or angled back, cut back or pull back to the UNMARKED team-mate or a team-mate moving away from his / her marker to latch on to the cross or pass in the opponent 18 yd / penalty area. During acceleration or retardation or change of direction of the winger with the ball – he / she must not over-hit or under-hit the ball – control, and the correct impact must be given to the ball by the player – utilise Newton's first law of motion for control.
Use 80% side-foot slide rule on the turf – fluent, silky smooth, one touch, unbroken well timed passes: and 20% long ball passes. Use long balls as an element of surprise ball.

On the turf passes are easier to control and made accurate, whereas long balls, especially over the top, are more difficult to control and usually go astray or to the opponent – they also give the opponent time and space to intercept. Remember – once you have created the chance, that is half of it – the other half is to implement the DEFINING MOMENT OF THE FINAL BALL past the opponent keeper. If you lose the ball during play double your effort to win the ball back and start a move again.
There are many additional goal-scoring ideas, which should help the players to score some fantastic goals – these are available on video-tape and digital versatile disc, players are advised to look at them from time to time which can be added to the training programme.

Goal Scoring Moves

Some examples of goal scoring moves are as follows – good SIGNALS from team-mate to team-mate.

(1) Winger can go it alone instead of going all the way down the flanks: move toward the opponent 18 yd box, zigzag through the path of least resistance with a good angle to side-foot the ball past the opponent keeper or pass or cut back to an UNMARKED team-mate.
Be careful of the tight angle area.

(2) Quick back-heel to an UNMARKED team-mate in a good striking position in the opponent 18 yd / penalty area.

(3) Side-foot, ball into the path of an UNMARKED team- mate in a good striking position.

(4) Solo zigzag dribble by a forward, "one on one" with the opponent keeper, send the keeper the wrong way or going around the keeper or chipping the keeper.

All goal scoring moves to be Perfect Practiced, so as to become automatic and instinctive – some moves to be statutory, and some to be changed from game to game, and week to week – this keeps the opponents guessing.

Style 2 Indirect - defence splitting –with a goal scoring move in mind

Consisting of strings of UNBROKEN side-foot slide rule on the turf, fluent, silky smooth, one touch, well timed, passes – a more indirect system to the opponent 18 yd / penalty area – using TWO TRICKY FLYING WINGERS and TWO TRICKY "HOLD UP" team-mates and the "FASTEST DRIBBLER".
From the moment of kick off on the centre circle pass to the left midfield team-mate then pass to the left winger – the right back, central defenders and left backs must stay in their positions to defend their goal, goalkeeper and goal area for 90 minutes plus extra time – remember to be prompted by the "QUEEN HORNET" and "QUEEN BEE" analogy the DEFINING MOMENT IN DEFENCE in the horizontal and vertical planes to keep a clean sheet.
If you use 3 / 4 defenders at the back – as play is pushed forward, one or two midfield team-mates may move forward to link up with the attack – while, one or two midfield team-mates fast back-track to fill the gaps left by the forward moving back 3 / 4 team-mates, the reason is, if you lose the ball and there is a quick break by the opponents, the two defending team-mates of the back 3 / 4 should be able to hold the fort till help arrives in the form of other defending team-mates, to close down, dispossess, clear or block off the opponents.
If at any time you happen to lose the ball during play – implement the DEFINING MOMENT IN DEFENCE, and win the ball back and start a move again. Bring Perfect Practice for set pieces into play when and where necessary during the 90 minutes plus extra time of the game.
Pass move and ride tackles quicker than the opponent – but you must also close down quicker than the opponent a STATUTORY MOVE.

Two tricky "HOLD UP" team-mates to get in the opponent 18 yd / penalty area and hold on to the ball, by shielding it – holding it – keeping it by applying his / her natural skills, such as dummy opponents – turning opponents – zigzag dribbling past opponents – teasing opponents – step-over – send opponents the wrong way, and then look up for his/her UNMARKED team-mate in splendid isolation to lay the ball in his / her path, and to set up chances for other team-mates to implement the DEFINING MOMENT OF THE FINAL BALL in either plane - or going all the way on his own to score.
If one "HOLD UP" team-mate becomes heavily marked by the opponents, then switch to the other one or substitute one and bring on another who is just as good. Bring the "FASTEST DRIBBLER" into play.

Look for the path of least resistance or least congested channel and use side-foot slide rule on the turf – fluent, silky smooth, one touch, unbroken, well timed passes to UNMARKED team-mates: look up and pass the ball to a midfield team-mate or directly to a right winger or left winger, pass and move, accelerate or decelerate or change direction, as the player see fit. The winger using the flanks very often runs at opponents, dribbling past them – holding, shielding the ball, making sure that well timed UNMARKED supports have arrived in the opponent 18 yd / penalty area: weave into their play the defence splitting side-foot slide rule on the turf – free flowing, delightful, fluent, silky smooth, one touch, unbroken, well timed intricate, angular and triangular, inter-passing and interchanging: and exchanging passes.
The following goal scoring moves described below to the UNMARKED team-mates, a "HOLD UP" team-mate, who can dribble with good ball control and ball skill, should be in the opponent 18 yd / penalty area, holding the ball and then laying the ball into the path of the UNMARKED team-mate to implement the DEFINING MOMENT OF THE FINAL BALL past the opponent keeper. TIMING, velocity, acceleration, retardation or change of direction between the wingers and his support team-mates have to be just right – too early or too late and a good created chance is wasted: the wingers and team-mates must not over-hit or under-hit the crosses or passes – the ball must be kicked or headed with the correct impact.
Once the chance is created by the wingers or team-mates to the UNMARKED team-mate who then converts the chance by implementing the DEFINING MOMENT OF THE FINAL BALL with feet or head past the opponent keeper either in the horizontal plane – horizontal to vertical, that is surface to air or the vertical plane. Persistent interplay in the opponent 18 / penalty area causes many problems for the opponents.

Use 80% side-foot slide rule on the turf – fluent, silky smooth, one touch, unbroken, well timed passes: and 20% long ball passes. Use long balls as an element of surprise ball. On the turf passes are easier to control and made accurate, whereas long balls, especially over the top, are more difficult to control and usually go astray or to the opponent.
Once you have created the chance, that is half of it – the other half is to implement the DEFINING MOMENT OF THE FINAL BALL past the opponent keeper. If you lose the ball during play, double your effort to win the ball back and quickly restart your moves again – this process is STATUTORY.

There are some additional goal scoring moves, which should help the forwards to score some fantastic goals – these are available on video tapes/DVD. The coach or manager will have some goal scoring ideas, which can be added to the training programme and weave into this style.

Goal Scoring Moves

Some examples of goal scoring moves are as follows – good SIGNALS from team-mate to team-mate.

(1) Side-foot slide rule pass from the "HOLD UP" team-mate into the path of an UNMARKED team-mate in the opponent 18 yd / penalty area to score.

(2) Side-foot slide rule pass from by team-mate to an UNMARKED team-mate in a good striking position in the opponent 18 yd / penalty area to score.

(3) A side-foot slide rule on the turf CUT BACK pass from a winger to an UNMARKED

team-mate in total isolation - in the opponent 18 yd / penalty area to score.

(4) Latch on to crosses from wingers into the opponent 18 yd / penalty area to an UNMARKED team-mate to head into goal or knock down for a scramble to score.

(5) Chest down a parabolic cross, line up and volley it past the opponent keeper to score Fig. 1 - 10

(6) Quick neat back-heel to an UNMARKED team-mate in the opponent 18 yd / penalty area to score.

(7) Glancing header from crosses coming into the opponent 18 yd / penalty area to an UNMARKED team-mate to score.

(8) Team-mate runs with the ball, at an angle towards the opponent goal, at the same time, another of his / her team-mate follows in his path – UNMARKED, and a few metres behind: the team-mate with the ball, then makes a quick neat back-heel to the following UNMARKED team-mate to side-foot past the opponent keeper to score – see co-ordinated back-heel in Chapter 8.

All goal scoring moves to have Perfect Practice, so as to become automatic and instinctive – some moves to be statutory, and some to be changed from game to game, and week to week – this keeps the opponents guessing and makes it difficult for them to know what you are going to do next.

Chest Down a Ball - eyes on the ball to the point of strike before ball hits turf

Fig. 1 – 10 team-mate makes a parabolic cross from the edge of the opponent 18 yd / box to an unmarked team-mate inside the opponent 18 yd box in splendid isolation to control a chest down, while he / she swivels on the right foot to implement the DEFINING MOMENT OF THE FINAL BALL with the left foot.

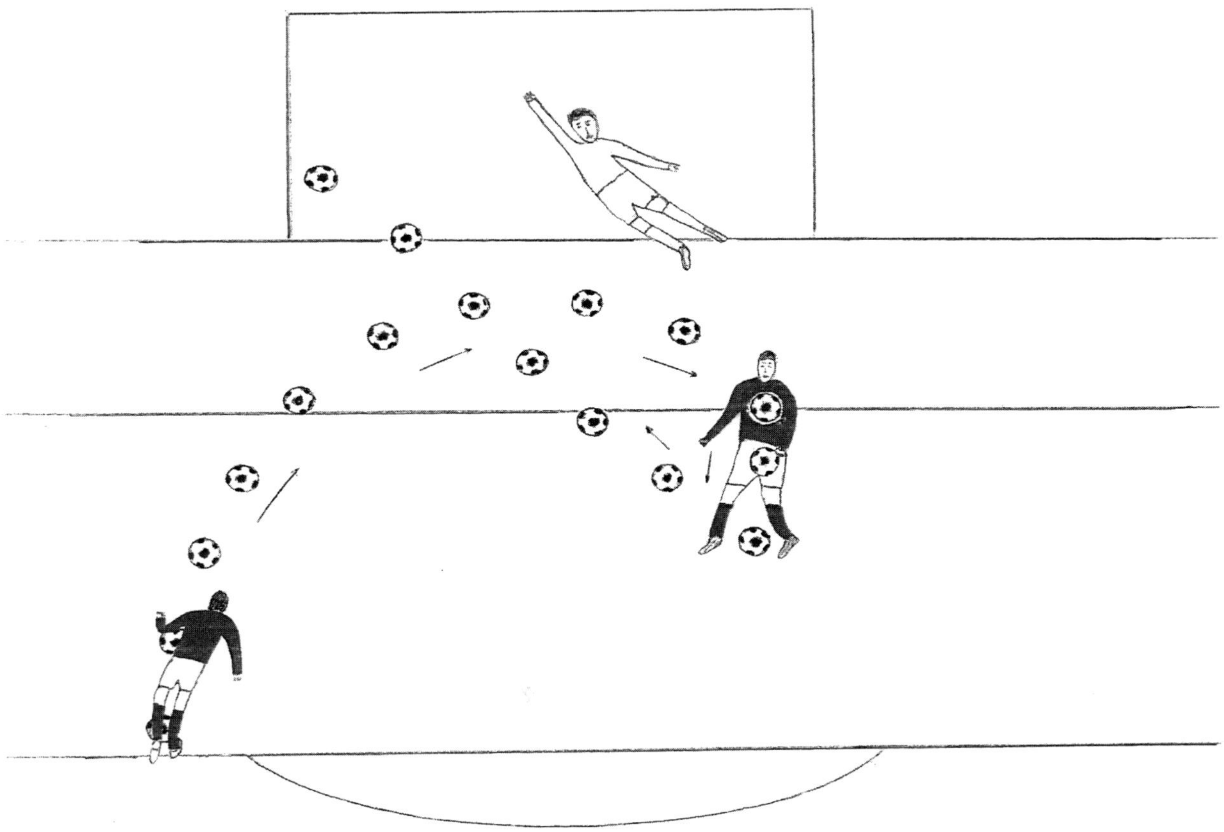

Style 3 – Switching Formations during Play with a goal scoring move in mind

Using a switching formation of (3 – 4 – 3) to (3 – 2 – 5) - and vice-versa during in-play.
The formation 3 – 4 – 3 is used for solid defending in your own half and when your team builds an attacking move you switch quickly to the formidable(3 – 2 – 5) attacking formation in the opponent 18 yd / penalty area – using TWO TRICKY FLYING WINGERS and quick intelligent back-track.
The forward support team-mate is like the inside right or inside left team-mate linking up with the wingers. Consisting of few side-foot slide rule on the turf, fluent, silky smooth, one touch unbroken well timed passes and crosses - a more direct system to the opponent 18 yd / penalty area.

From the moment of kick off – the right back, central defenders and left backs must stay in their positions to defend their goal, goalkeeper and goal area for 90 minutes plus extra time – remember to be prompted by the "QUEEN HORNET" and "QUEEN BEE" analogy the DEFINING MOMENT IN DEFENCE in the horizontal and vertical planes to keep a clean sheet.
With 3 defenders at the back, as play is pushed forward, one defender may move forward to link up with up with the attack, while one midfield team-mate fast back-track to fill the gaps left by the forward moving back 3 team-mate, the reason is, if you lose the ball and there is a quick break by the opponents, the two defending team-mates of the back 3 should be able to hold the fort till help arrives in the form of other defending team-mates, to close down, dispossess, clear or block off the opponents. Intelligent back-tracking - quick reaction and response are a must.
If at any time you happen to lose the ball during play – implement the DEFINING MOMENT IN DEFENCE, and win the ball back and start a move again. Bring Perfect Practice for set pieces into play when – and where necessary during the 90 minutes plus extra time of the game.

Pass, and move and ride tackles quicker than the opponent – but you must also close down quicker than the opponent – A STATUTORY MOVE.

Taking the path of least resistance, the wingers using the flanks very often, receives slide rule passes from the back 3 or midfield team-mates, runs at the opponents, gets past or behind them, to get the cross or pass across the face of the opponent goal: while at the same time – the two ROVING midfield team-mates link up with the centre forward in unmarked positions to give support to the wingers in the opponent 18 yd / penalty area to implement the DEFINING MOMENT OF THE FINAL BALL.
So, in attack you can have 5 forwards in the opponent 18 yd / penalty area – but, also ready to back-track and double your effort to win the ball back, just in case you lose possession: a clean sheet a priority and scoring goals a must.
Use 80% side-foot slide rule on the turf – fluent, silky smooth, one touch, unbroken, well timed passes: and 20% long ball passes. Use long balls as an element of surprise ball.
On the turf passes are easier to control and made accurate, whereas long balls, especially over the top, are more difficult to control and usually go astray or to the opponent.
Once you have created the chance, that is half of it – the other half is to implement the DEFINING MOMENT OF THE FINAL BALL past the opponent keeper. If you lose the ball during play, double your effort to win the ball back and quickly restart your move.
There are some additional goal scoring moves, which should help the forwards to score some fantastic goals – these are available on video tapes/DVD. The coach or manager will have some goal scoring ideas, which can be added to the training programme.

Goal Scoring Moves –

Some examples of goal scoring moves are as follows – good SIGNALS from team-mate to team-mate

Slide rule cross from either winger to an UNMARKED team-mate in and around the opponent 18 yd / penalty area to implement an instinctive slide rule strike past the keeper to score.

(1) Set up an UNMARKED team–mate in splendid isolation with a delightful one – two slide rule, exchanging passes in the opponent 18yd/ penalty area to score.

(2) Slide rule cut back from either winger to an UNMARKED team-mate in the opponent 18 yd / penalty area to score.

(3) Chest down the ball for slide rule control, line up – then slide rule volley past the opponent keeper to score.

(4) A spectacular slide rule diving header – from a winger's slide rule cross to an UNMARKED team-mate in the opponent 18 yd / penalty area to score.

(5) Back heel: team-mate back heel's to an UNMARKED team-mate some metres behind who then side-foot slide rule the ball past the opponent keeper to score.

(6) A 25–30 yd / m., dipping strike that lands on the turf just in front or out of reach of the opponent keeper to score.

(7) UNMARKED team-mate receives the ball in the opponent 18 yd / penalty area - controls it - flicks it upward – juggles the ball with both feet for a few moments, if time and space are available then implement a slide rule volley past the opponent keeper to score.

(8) Individual effort – persistent solo dribbling by naturally gifted team-mate to dribble past opponents to score – the "FASTEST DRIBBLER" in action.

All goal scoring moves to be Perfect Practiced, so as to become automatic and instinctive – some moves to be statutory - and some to be changed from game to game, and week to week – this keeps the opponents guessing.

Another option that can be added to this 3 – 2 – 5 system – is one attacking move is doubled up – that is, if a right winger runs down the flank with the ball – at the same time his / her inside right team-mate runs parallel with the winger – say 5 metres apart to exchange passes to implement the DEFINING MOMENT OF THE FINAL BALL by latching on to a cross, a pass or a cut back from the winger in the opponent 18 yd / penalty area: this is well suited to use two "FASTEST DRIBBLERS" on this occasion.
The left winger could do the same with his / her inside left team-mate, when the chance is created.

Style 4 – Naturally Gifted Players with a goal scoring move in mind

This style consists of few side-foot slide rule on the turf, fluent, silky smooth, one touch, unbroken well timed passes: a quick direct path of least resistance to the opponent 18 yd / penalty area using TWO TRICKY FLYING WINGERS, and TWO or THREE "HOLD UP" team-mates and the fastest dribbler. From the moment of kick off the two team-mates on the centre circle pass to each other and move forward then pass to either winger who is also moving forward – the right back, central defenders and left backs must stay in their positions to defend their, goalkeeper and goal area for 90 minutes plus extra time – remember to be prompted by the "QUEEN HORNET" and "QUEEN BEE" analogy- the DEFINING MOMENT IN DEFENCE in the horizontal and vertical planes to keep a CLEAN SHEET.
If you use 3 / 4 defenders at the back, as play is pushed forward, one defender may move forward to link up with up with the attack, while one midfield team-mate fast back-track to fill the gaps left by the forward moving back 3 / 4 team-mates, the reason is, if you lose the ball and there is a quick break by the opponents, the two defending team-mates of the back 3 / 4should be able to hold the fort till help arrives in

the form of other defending team-mates to close down, dispossess, clear or block off the opponents. Intelligent fast back-tracking quick reaction and response must be automatic and instinctive.
If at any time you happen to lose the ball during play – implement the DEFINING MOMENT IN DEFENCE, and win the ball back and start a move again. Bring Perfect Practice for set pieces into play when – and where necessary during the 90 minutes plus extra time of the game.

Pass, and move and ride tackles quicker than the opponent – but you must also close down quicker than the opponent – A STATUTORY MOVE.

The TWO or THREE "HOLD UP" team-mates in the opponent 18 yd / penalty area to hold on to the ball, by shielding it – holding it – keeping it by applying his / her natural skills and tricks such as to dummy opponents, turn opponents – send opponents the wrong way and look up for his / her UNMARKED team-mate in splendid isolation to lay the ball in his / her path – linking up with other "HOLD UP" team-mates, and set up chances for other team-mates to implement the DEFINING MOMENT OF THE FINAL BALL. If one "HOLD UP" player becomes heavily marked by the opponents, then switch the work load to the other one or two or substitute one and bring on another who is just as good – remember when substitutions are made the optimum standard of play must not fall. These "hold up" players - dominates attention during play.

Perfect Practice on the training ground, and implement on match days.

This style is based on 10 players in the team who have natural gifts in DEFENCE and ATTACK – ball control – passing – possession – and the DEFINING MOMENT OF THE FINAL BALL – and must include two tricky wingers. The goalkeeper to help co-ordinate and organise the defence around his / her goal area – watch out for UNMARKED OPPONENTS in dangerous areas, and remind his / her defenders to CLOSE DOWN the opponents quickly and safely.
These high calibre naturally gifted players with the ability to read the game during play, and under pressure – good anticipation with his / her team-mates, and to anticipate what the opponents are going to do – for example to intercept a dangerous cross or pass from the opponent and to start to build an attacking move. To use the fluid and particle dynamics discussed in this manual to enhance their game to an even higher level. Perform mesmerising tricks with the ball, and run at the opponent defence. To accelerate, decelerate or change direction, as is necessary – to dummy the opponent – juggling with the ball – running at defenders: sending opponents the wrong way – turning defenders – attracting the ball like a magnet to their feet: running rings round the opponent to keep the ball – UNBROKEN SLIDE RULE PASSES: look up – pass and move to UNMARKED team-mate to team-mate who can do the same to keep possession.
This is an exciting style to play by, but it will be difficult to find 10 naturally gifted players to fit into any team for various reasons – if the coach or manager could get 50% of the gifted players in his / her team, he / she will certainly have a team that will play good exciting football. Perform tricks with the ball, and run at the opponent defence – make them back–pedal to confusion.
This style could be slotted into styles 1 – 2 or 3 depending on the choice of the coach or manager. Use 80% side-foot slide rule on the turf, fluent, silky smooth, one touch, unbroken, well timed passes: and 20% long ball. Use long balls as an element of surprise ball. On the turf passes are easier to control, and made accurate, whereas long balls, especially over the top, are more difficult to control, and almost always go astray or to the opponent. Be ready to back-track, and double your effort to win the ball back, just in case you lose possession – a CLEAN SHEET a priority, and scoring goals a must.

Remember - once you have created the chance, that is half of it – other half is to implement the DEFINING MOMENT OF THE FINAL BALL past the opponent keeper. If you lose the ball during play, double your effort to win back the ball, and quickly restart your move again.
There are some additional goal scoring moves, which should help the forwards to score some fantastic goals – these are available on videotapes and DVD. The coach or manager will have some goal scoring ideas, which can be added to the training programme.

Goal Scoring Moves

Some examples of goal scoring moves are as follows – good SIGNALS from team-mate to team-mate.

(1) An over the top slide rule pass from the back 3 / 4 to the UNMARKED centre forward, to place the ball past the opponent keeper to score.

(2) Slide rule cut back from either winger to an UNMARKED team-mate in the opponent 18 yd / penalty area to score.

(3) Set up an UNMARKED team-mate with a delightful one-two slide rule, exchanging passes in the opponent 18 yd / penalty area to score.

(4) Receiving a slide rule cross from a winger, and chipping the opponent keeper with a slide rule chip, especially, if the keeper is off his / her line.

(5) A 25–30 yd, dipping strike that lands on the turf just in front or out of reach of the opponent keeper to score.

(6) A spectacular slide rule diving header – from a winger's slide rule cross to an UNMARKED team-mate in the opponent 18 yd / penalty area to score.

(7) Feeding an UNMARKED team-mate in the opponent 18 yd / penalty area, with a slide rule square pass from either flanks to score.

(8) Nodding a slide rule cross into the opponent 18 yd / penalty area to an UNMARKED team-mate to implement a slide rule volley past the opponent keeper to score.

(9) Sideways scissors strike, Fig. 4-8

All goal scoring moves to be Perfect Practiced, so as to become automatic, and instinctive – some moves to be statutory, and some to be changed from game to game, and week to week, this keeps the opponents guessing as to what you are going to do next.

When things go wrong in Football / Soccer

Examples of – How to put them Right

Check out and correct

When you lose a game this means that you have done something or a combination of things wrong: sometimes the referee may be at fault – but referees are circumstances beyond your control.

When you lose game after game, then you are repeating your mistakes, and this could make the team chaotic and dysfunctional, are you using the correct combinations of team-mates in a game for instance?
Where do you start to put things right? Look for inherent faults in training and playing.

The coach or manager has to assess, and analyse the problems, then find solutions to these problems – ask deep searching questions: most of the answers are in this manual.

Start by going back to basics – make sure that 4 dependant variables, ball control – passing – possession and the DEFINING MOMENT OF THE FINAL BALL are all up to standard of this manual.

This is the solid base to start from, and put right, and this is statutory: then look at other problems like the DEFENCE and ATTACK.
Check out the standard of the particular style used from styles 1 – 2 - 3 - & 4.

Check out the dynamics of play – high number of bad passes made by a player - reduce to a low number.

Watch how the players perform during training, and on match days. Look at videotapes or DVD of the last game or previous games – check out for faults – carefully in slow motion. Check out each department of play in detail. Check out for lack of goal scoring opportunity SIGNALS from team-mate to team-mate. Arms up.

Check out every angle – mental and physical aspects.
Check out each player individually, including the goalkeeper.
Check out the coach or manager, and other members of the training staff for malfunction.

Check out for HIDDEN DANGERS as given in this manual.

Check out all aspects of the defence – the understanding, and co-ordination between defenders, and the goalkeeper helping each other, and watching for each other – at all times during the 90 – minutes plus extra time of play.

When you lose the ball – quickness of the reaction and response, and check out that defenders are implementing the DEFINING MOMENT IN DEFENCE – this is where defenders are prompted to mark tightly and close down the opponents in pairs or three's quickly, fairly, and decisively – dispossessing the opponents in numbers.

Check out for decisive clearances by defenders in dangerous areas.
Check out that defenders are intercepting the opponent passes before the opponent can get into a dangerous area. Hesitant - lack of discipline, sloppy defending and chasing shadows.

Not closing down the UNMARKED opponent quickly. Correct by speeding up.

Poor wall set up in relation to the team's goalkeeper - when defending a free kick in a dangerous area.

Check out for players BALL WATCHING – not challenging for the ball – lapse in marking.

Slow back-tracking by defenders who go forward.

Total backing off by team defenders and no challenges made for the ball.

Fear factor – check out and correct.

Critical times lapse in concentration during play – check out and correct.

Not defending or attacking for 90 minutes plus extra time of play.

Drop in energy level – body language.

Not pressurising the opponents for 90 minutes plus extra time.

Not following instructions given by the coach or manager.

Over the top celebration when goals are scored – check and correct by reducing.

Player's life styles in relation to fitness, and team's performance – late night partying, and alcohol abuse before games - troublemakers – check out and correct. Unsettled players want to leave – let them go.

Show character of players when goals are conceded – lack of consolidation, how to come back.

Sitting back after scoring – check out and correct – by scoring more goals.
Not consolidating lead and position – check out and correct.

Intimidation and provocation by the opponents – check out and correct by walking away – show character, and good sense. Getting caught up in media propaganda and hype – ignore.

Coping with pressure – do what is right – get it right – keep it right.
These are some of the things that can go wrong for a team, and usually leads to lack of confidence – consistency – and continuity – but by knowing EXACTLY what to look for, and correcting early: serious, and long term problems can be avoided- there are many other things that can go wrong for a team, and it is the responsibility of the coach or manager to put things right, more examples –

Is the team implementing the – FLUID and PARTICLE DYNAMICS facilities with optimum efficiency?

Is the team passing and moving QUICKER than the opponent?

Is the team implementing the "DEFINING MOMENT IN DEFENCE" with optimum efficiency?

Is the team giving away too many free kicks in dangerous areas?

Is the team implementing the DEFINING MOMENT OF THE FINAL BALL with optimum efficiency?

Is the team implementing the SET PIECES with optimum efficiency?

Is the team leaking goals and not scoring over a number of games – check out and correct.

The Referee and Referee Assistance

The referee standard varies from referee to referee, assistants to assistants, and match to match, but in general it is quite good, considering some of the split – second decisions, they have to make under difficult conditions at times. Sometimes a referee or assistants makes the wrong decision, and this causes upset to one team, and occasionally to both teams – trying to sort out who is right and who is wrong for various reasons can be quite difficult at times.
A good idea to help the referee and assistants to get a true, and conclusive answer to tight decisions is to install the HAWK EYE type of cameras that are used in the cricket stumps which picks up close up of tight umpiring decisions, relayed back to the third umpire in the stand, and the result flashed on a big screen for all to see. If these cameras are conveniently placed in the goal posts, they will be able to zoom in at different angles, to tell whether the ball has crossed the line or not.
The same should be done with regards to tight offside decisions, where cameras are placed near the roof of the stand along the length of the pitch, so as to zoom in to tight offside decisions – the pitch referee could then refer to the third camera referee for the final decision which is flashed on to the big screen for everyone to see. This idea may not suit every club, because of the expense.
Objects thrown on the pitch should not be allowed – they may have a hand in the result and this makes it invalid. There are some books that give explanations on the rules of football / soccer, and players are advised to revise them and note when changes are made in order not to break them.

TO WIN GAMES – POINTS AND TROPHIES the
following must be at the highest standard.
Be even "more up for it" than the opponent

PREPARATION is the mental, and
physical Perfect Practice
in all departments of play –
on the training ground.

Being READY– is the ability to
implement the PREPARATION
on match days with
optimum performance.
So, ask yourselves –
ARE YOU PREPARED?
BUT
ARE YOU READY?

Good Luck!

* 9 7 8 1 7 8 0 3 5 4 4 1 5 *

SD - #0067 - 140926 - C0 - 297/210/9 - PB - 9781780354415 - Gloss Lamination